MEDITERRANEAN DIET

A day-to-day guide for keeping yourself genetically young

By

ISAIAH TOLU OYERINOLA

This report is towards furnishing precise and solid data concerning the point and issue secured. The production is sold with the possibility that the distributor isn't required to render bookkeeping, formally allowed, or something else, qualified administrations. On the off chance that exhortation is important, lawful, or proficient, a rehearsed individual in the calling ought to be requested.

The Declaration of Principles, which was also recognized and endorsed by the Committee of the American Bar Association and the Committee of Publishers and Associations.

The data gave in this is expressed, to be honest, and predictable, in that any risk, as far as absentmindedness or something else, by any utilization or maltreatment of any approaches, procedures, or bearings contained inside is the singular and articulate obligation of the beneficiary peruser. By no means will any lawful obligation or fault be held against the distributor for any reparation, harms, or money related misfortune because of the data in this, either straightforwardly or by implication.

Particular creators claim all copyrights not held by the distributor.

The data in this is offered for educational purposes exclusively and is all-inclusive as so. The introduction of the data is without a contract or any sort of assurance confirmation.

The trademarks that are utilized are with no assent, and the distribution of the trademark is without consent or support by the trademark proprietor. All trademarks and brands inside this book are for explaining purposes just and are simply possessed by the proprietors, not partnered with this record.

Disclaimer

All the material contained in this book is provided for educational and informational purposes only. No responsibility can be taken for any results or outcomes resulting from the use of this material. While every attempt has been made to provide information that is both accurate and effective, the author does not assume any responsibility for the accuracy or use/misuse of the information herein.

Table of Contents

INTRODUCTION 10

CHAPTER ONE: HISTORY OF MEDITTERANEAN DIET PLAN 13

CHAPTER TWO: WHAT IS MEDITERRANEAN DIET PLAN? 22

CHAPTER THREE: COMMON MISTAKES AND MYTHS THAT SABOTAGE THE MEDITERRANEAN DIET 32

CHAPTER FOUR: HEALTH AND MEDICAL BENEFITS OF A MEDITERRANEAN FOOD DIET 40

CHAPTER FIVE: MEDITERRANEAN BREAKFAST 49

1.   Caprese Avocado Toast 49

2.   Bacon-Avocado 49

3.   THE CAULIFLOWER CARBONARA PAN MEAL 50

4.   FLAXSEED CRACKERS 50

5.   HEALTHFUL CHICKEN SALAD 50

Everyone needs the right amount of healthy fat to stay alive and be healthy. This Mediterranean meal gives you the required protein and fat that you need. To make this meal you must have in your possession, 2 cups of Chicken breast pieces, 2 cups of cut steamed green beans, 1/2 cup of homemade mayonnaise, 1/2 cup of diced pecans, 1/4 cup of diced cilantro, 1/4 cup of basil leaves, 1/4 cup of mint leaves, 1/2 tablespoon salt and 1/2 tablespoon of white pepper. See chapter 12 for detailed cooking instruction. 50

6.   Eggs with Zucchini, Summer Tomatoes, and a sprinkle of Bell Peppers 51

7.   Poached Egg added to crisp White Beans or Green Bean 51

8.   Hazelnuts, Blueberries, and Lemon with Grain Salad for Mediterranean Breakfast 52

9.   Chilled or refrigerated Wraps of Spinach Feta for Mediterranean Breakfast 52

10.   Avocado and Egg Breakfast Pizza 52

11.   Spinach Artichoke Frittata for Mediterranean Breakfast 53

12.   Healthy Fruit Salad for Mediterranean Breakfast...................53

13.   Mediterranean Breakfast Pita...53

14.   Easy Muesli for Breakfast..53

15.   Opt for whole-grain bread. 54

16.   English muffin with high nutritious toppings.......................54

17.   Yogurt drizzle with a small honey 55

CHAPTER SIX: MEDITERRANEAN LUNCH...56

1.   Lemony Orzo Salad 56

2.   Cauli Rice, And Chicken Cutlet...57

3.   Shirataki Noodles (Konjac)And Asian Salad............................57

4.   Falafel Kale Salad with Tahini Dressing....................................58

5.   Lettuce Meal 58

6.   GRILLED COD AND SHRIMPS...58

7.   Gluten-Free Mediterranean Pasta 59

8.   Classic Mediterranean Salad...59

9.   Mediterranean Lentil Salad..60

10.   Greek Turkey Meatball Gyro with Tzatziki..............................60

11.   A bowl of Mediterranean Pepper Sauce that is well roasted
With Quinoa 61

12.   Greek Shrimp Souvlaki and Farro Bowl..................................61

13.   Greek Lemon Chicken Soup 61

14.   Lemon Parmesan Chicken with Zucchini Noodles 62

15.   Quinoa Stuffed Eggplant with Tahini Sauce...........................62

16.   Bulgar Salad with Feta..62

17.   Mediterranean Veggie Sandwich...63

CHAPTER SEVEN: MEDITERRANEAN DINNER...................................64

1.   Greek-Style Baked Cod with Lemon and Garlic 64

2.   Arugula Salad With Basil Vinaigrette................................. 64

3.   BROCCOLI AND ROSEMARY CHICKEN 65

4.   Kale Beef and Vegetables Wrapped In Avocado and Olive Oil . 65

5.   Mushroom and Broccoli and Bacon Meal 65

6.   Garlic and Lemon with Greek-Style Baked Cod 66

7.   Chicken Shawarma... 66

8.   Moroccan Vegetable Tagine 67

9.   Easy Seafood Paella.. 67

10.   Spanakopita 67

11.   Chicken Souvlaki 68

12.   Briam 68

13.   Grilled Kofta Kebabs.. 69

14.   Italian Baked Chicken 69

15.   Moroccan Lamb Stew 69

16.   Falafel 70

17.   Shakshuka 70

CHAPTER EIGHT: MEDITERRANEAN DESSERT 71

1.   Italian Apple Olive Oil Cake.. 71

2.   Low Carb Bread 72

3.   THE MEDITERRANEAN ALMOND BUTTER BURGER 72

4.   ASPARAGUS, SAUCE AND AVOCADO BOAT MEAL 73

5.   SESAME SALAD AND CHICKEN BROCHETTES 73

6.   Popped Quinoa Crunch Bar.. 73

7.   Honey Almond Ricotta Spread with Peaches........................ 74

8.   Blueberry Muffins for dessert....................................... 74

9.   Flourless Chocolate Olive Oil Cake................................. 75

10.   Healthy Energy Bites 75

11.   Roasted Fruit 76

12.   Whole Grain Citrus and Olive Oil Muffins 76

13.   Vegan Lemon Olive Oil Cake 76

14.   Pistachio No-Bake Snack Bars 77

15.   Maple Vanilla Baked Pears.. 77

16.   Olive Oil Chocolate Chip Cookies 78

17.   Fig Almond Olive Oil Cake 78

CHAPTER NINE: MEDITERRANEAN SNACKS 80

1.   Mediterranean Thin Crust Flatbread 80

2.   CHICKEN GRILLED THIGH WITH ZUCCHINI SALAD..... 81

3.   GRILLED SALMON AND GREEN BEANS AND RADISHES 81

4.   MEDITERRANEAN BAKED OMELET 81

5.   Smoked Salmon Goat Cheese Endive Bites.................. 82

6.   15-Minute Mediterranean Chickpea Salad 83

7.   Loaded Mediterranean Hummus................................... 83

8.   Crock-Pot Chunky Monkey Paleo Trail Mix 84

9.   Smoky Loaded Eggplant Dip.. 84

10.   Peanut Butter Banana Greek Yogurt Bowl 85

11.   Mediterranean Roasted Chickpeas............................... 85

12.   Savory Feta Spinach and Sweet Red Pepper Muffins 86

13.   Baked Whole-Grain Lavash Chips and Mediterranean Dip.... 86

14.   7-Ingredient Quinoa Granola 87

15.   Greek Yogurt Spinach Artichoke Dip............................. 87

16.   Smoked Salmon, Avocado, and Cucumber Bites 88

17.   Whole-Wheat Banana Blueberry Muffins...................... 88

CHAPTER TEN: VEGAN ALTERNATIVES 90

1.   Prioritize omega-three fatty acids 91

2.   Be clever about your diet and take the right amount of protein intake 93

3.   Go for variety 93

CHAPTER ELEVEN: MEDITERRANEAN FOODS, EXERCISE, NUTRITION AND THEIR CONTRIBUTION TO LONGEVITY AND EXCITING LIFESPAN 99

1.   The Basic of Longevity...100

2.   The Best Exercise Routine for Longevity When You Are Observing Mediterranean Diet 103

Walk fast for an hour every day..103

Cardiovascular exercise for 2.5 to 5 hours per week.....................103

Use Mediterranean diet, weight exercises or weightless exercises to strengthen all your muscles..104

3.   Energy Production...105

4.   Pro and Cons of Mediterranean Diet When Not Done in Proper Proportion 108

CHAPTER TWELVE: A WEEKLY PLAN OF MEDITERRANEAN DIET 111

1.   First Week 111

2.   Second Week 149

3.   Third Week..191

4.   Fourth Week 228

CONCLUSION..264

INTRODUCTION

It is more of an open secret that someone who loves looking good and wants to experience a good life would be interested in whatever goes into his or her mouth. I believe that presupposes that such an individual would be full of skepticism about some foods and at the same time would have a very inquisitive mind of the highest order to ask the necessary question about the rationale behind this book been titled: *"The Mediterranean diet meal prep: healthy recipes for lasting weight loss and 4 weeks meal plan."* Well, if before buying this book or before taking it from the bookshelf, bookstore or library you had done yourself good by posing that critical yet harmless question, I would like to share a piece of great news with you. Congratulations, you are about to have your heart desires and realize your dream of losing weight, detoxifying your body through proper application of Mediterranean food! Even though there are no bad news but only the good ones, the good news that I would like to share with you is that you are almost at the finish line of achieving your dream body and having an elongated lifestyle.

What I am saying is that by having this book in your hands, you are already halfway to the finish line on your journey to detoxify yourself, lose weight, promote your muscle growth, gain longevity and prevent preventable disease which can cost you a fortune to control if not properly taken care of in time. The fact is this book is loaded with a series of affordable recipes that will promote your health and wellbeing. By choosing this book, you have already started your journey to educate your mind and have real knowledge and understanding of Mediterranean diet. The book will lay bare the needed information which will help you in determining and choosing your lifestyle and understand what you eat. This book also contains information that will help you to maintain the faultless body; younger look, it will help you shed unnecessary weight and will show you how you can remain fit at all time through the Mediterranean foods. This book has also been written to help you in choosing what to consume, when to consume them and what to avoid and when to avoid them; it will also help you maintain a healthy lifestyle; it will also shape your mind and eventually give you sound mind and vision, and body and at the same time. The book is also designed to show you how you can cook your food at home and save costs – if the information in this book are followed religiously, you will definitely have a body that betrays your age – or what do you think about having a young body even at the old age.

As you begin to read this book, I want you to open your mind and understand that living for a long time does not necessarily mean living well and longevity does not automatically translate into quality of life. How satisfying is it to live for a long time without truly living to your fullest abilities and capabilities? To have a long-life, free of health complications, you must eat some certain foods and that is what this book is out to explain to you.

Having longevity through proper observation of Mediterranean recipes is best experienced in a context that includes the best health characteristics: energy, vitality, physical strength and primary strength.   And beyond those dimensions of health, others illuminate well-being: positive moods, self-confidence, cognitive clarity, creativity, and self-realization which are realizable through consumption of the Mediterranean diet and proportionate intake of green leaves and seafood. Even more, there are states of being that are called transcendent, which belong to the highest levels of self-expression. The transcendent states are the road to a healthier mental strength. All these aspects of health are related and intertwined, and interactive with the Mediterranean foods. Improvement in any part of your body has a chain effect on every part of your body. Therefore, this book has sufficiently captured all the needed information that will help you in living a good, long and sickness free life through the application of Mediterranean diets. Lastly, there is a chapter that is solely written about the food you should eat and how to prepare them – this is to help you to cut costs, and the same time, eat right and live a healthy life.

CHAPTER ONE: HISTORY OF MEDITTERANEAN DIET PLAN

The History of the Mediterranean food culture can be said to cross many countries and I will do justice to it in this book. The linear yet long chronicle of the Mediterranean cuisines or diet plan is interesting and yet cannot be discussed without crossing and mentioning different cultures which eventually led to the food culture that we now call the Mediterranean diet.

The Mediterranean food plan has its origins in a portion of land considered specific in its kind, the Mediterranean Sea, which historians call "the cradle of society", due to the fact that inside its geographical borders, the whole records of the historic world can be said to have begun.

Mediterranean ocean, at its banks, stretched the valley of the Nile, the web of a historical and advanced civilization, and the exquisite seas of the Tigris and Euphrates, which have been the surroundings of the culture of the Sumerians, Assyrians, Babylonians, and Persians. In the Mediterranean location begun the energy of the Cretans, then emerged the Phoenicians and the founding of Greeks and their culture as much as the emerging strength of Rome, which allowed the territory to turn out to be the "accurate land" between the East and the West. From that time, the Mediterranean has become the meeting location of human beings who, with their contacts, have once in a while modified cultures, customs, languages, religions, and ways of thinking about reworking and converting lifestyle with the development of history. The clash of these ancient cultures produced what we can term partial integration; therefore, the food habit, diet, cuisines and their customs can be said to almost be the same in the past.

The origins of the "Mediterranean Diet" have been lost in the passage of time due to the fact that they got lost into the food eating customs and tradition of the Middle Ages, where in the ancient Roman lifestyle - the real version of the Greek – is known for its bread, wine and oil products which is basically the symbol of rural tradition and agriculture or agrarian society (and symbols chosen for the brand new faith which emerged then), supplemented by sheep cheese, vegetables (leeks, mallow, lettuce, chicory, mushrooms), little meat and a strong choice for fish and seafood (of which historical Rome turned into very gluttonous) are all what defined the Mediterranean cuisine or diet. The rich classes cherished the fresh fish (those aristocrats ate normally fried foods, well dipped in olive oil or grilled) and seafood oysters, consuming uncooked or fried. Slaves of Rome, however, become made to eat bad food which consists of bread and 1/2 a pound of wheat and olive oil a month, with some salted fish, not often a slice of touch meat is included in their food. The Roman way of life quickly clashed with the style of meals imported from the subculture of the German peoples, especially nomads, living in close harmony with the forest, derived from the same, with hunting, farming and gathering, maximum of the meal's resources. Pigs that were raised for their fats were broadly used in the kitchen to make their food. They also grew vegetables in small gardens near the camps. The few grains grown were now never used to make bread, but beer. The clash of those two cultures produced their partial integration so even their eating habits merged and become a fusion of new diet which is known as Mediterranean food. However, the Roman tradition distinct itself by being unwilling to trade the style of "The Mediterranean" feeding with that barbarian during this time. The critical elements of the Mediterranean food plan, that's the triad oil bread and wine had been exported alternatively in regions of the continent of Europe by the monastic orders, which migrated in one area of Europe and was used to evangelize and radicalize the other people's eating habit. Bread, oil and wine, have been, in fact, the central factors of the Christian liturgy; however, they had been later followed also in the eating habit of the common people of Europe. The new meals subculture was born from the union and the fusion of the dietary styles of two unique civilizations, the Christian Roman Empire and the German's. This culture later crossed borders with the passage of time, with a third lifestyle formed which was evident in the Arabian culture, which had advanced its very own unique food tradition at the southern seashores of the Mediterranean areas.

We can say Muslims gave a boost to a renewal of agriculture that encouraged the meals model with the introduction of plant species recognized or used in the Mediterranean foods. This was most effective and eaten among the wealthier social classes, due to the exorbitant and ridiculous prices that it was sold. It can be said to include sugar cane, rice, citrus, eggplant, spinach, and spices, as well as the newly discovered use delicacies of southern Europe, rose water, oranges, lemons, almonds, and pomegranates.

Islamic culture, therefore, participates within the trade and transformation of the cultural unity of the Mediterranean, which Rome had built, and provides a decisive contribution to the new culinary version that become the order of the day. An enormous variety of meals, exceeded by, dragging their preparation techniques and recipes among Greek in Europe and Muslim in Asians were also formed in the Mediterranean regions. Another event of outstanding historical effect was the discovery of America by the Europeans. This discovery is in, a way reflected in a "adoption" of some parts of the culinary way and customs, life and recent foodstuffs which includes potatoes, tomatoes, corn, peppers, and chili, as well as special varieties of beans which were also used. The tomato, "special curiosity", ornamental fruit is the most effective among them, it is recently taken into consideration as edible vegetables. This has later become the primary red vegetable that enriched the cuisine of Mediterranean but later became a perfect representation of the Mediterranean cuisine and it is now accepted as the Mediterranean diet by many people.

If the centrality of vegetables is one among the maximum original characters of the Mediterranean culture, it's far vital to consider the position of cereals as the one of the simple cooking and as a weapon of everyday survival, because of their "capability to fill" reducing hunger pangs of any nature. The formation of habits for cereals consumption, in addition to the modes of processing, assumes an exceptional part among the available foods. It was also used as the food which was used to differentiate areas and represents the geographical connotations and traditions that characterize the populations of the countries bordering on the Mediterranean Sea. Bread, polenta, couscous, soups, paella, and pasta are exclusive ways to eat cereals among the European during those periods.

This historical path just described and helped us figure out many similarities among the Mediterranean diet and the current eating diet of many people around the world. It illustrates the presence of an actual path that existed from the time of the eating habit of the ancient Egyptians to the discovery of America. This path can be assumed to be the only thing that led to the creation of new foods, giving us the Mediterranean diet weight loss diet plan that we know today.

The Mediterranean Diet is nutritional, and it is so universally favored by many people from different parts of the world. This makes it belongs to the cultural, historical, social, territorial and environmental items which can be used to tell people's story and origin. Also, it is closely associated with the way of life of the Mediterranean peoples throughout their history. The Candidature Dossier submitted to UNESCO by the special group asked to find out about the Mediterranean culture defines the Mediterranean Diet as follows:... Deriving from the Greek word "diaita"- way of life, - it is a social practice primarily based on all the "savoir-faire", knowledge, traditions ranging from the landscape to the desk and masking the Mediterranean Sea, cultures, harvesting, fishing, conservation, processing, preparation, cooking and especially the manner we eat the people associated with the Northern regions of Europe i.e., conviviality.

The Mediterranean diet, which is recognized basically as a food version, enhances the first-class taste, flavor and safety of each ingredient and shows their link to the land of origin. It gives an easy cuisine, however rich in look, very appealing and tastes way better, taking complete gain of all elements of healthful and rich food. It is an ethical desire that preserves the traditions and customs of the peoples of the Mediterranean area. Feeding can profoundly affect the health of an individual; this is because a good nutritional status enables one to keep a great degree of fitness and allows the prevention of metabolic diseases which include obesity, diabetes, hypertension, etc. The Mediterranean Diet is likewise an "aid for sustainable development. It is a meal that is very crucial for all the countries bordering on the Mediterranean. It is essential to the monastery and subculture impacts on food all over the world. In fact, the food covers all through the region and the capacity to inspire an experience of continuity and identity for local human beings are all that distinguish this diet.

Mediterranean weight loss plan: eating behaviors and lifestyles
The discovery of the health advantages of the Mediterranean Diet is attributed to the American scientist Ancel Keys of the University of Minnesota School of Power, which talked about the correlation between cardiovascular disease and weight loss plan for the first time. Ancel Keys, in the 50s, was so struck by a phenomenon, which he could not, at first, provide a full explanation. The terrible population of small cities of southern Italy turned into, against all predictions, much healthier than the rich citizens of New York, either of their personal households who emigrated in many decades ago to the United States are also used in the research. Keys advised

that these trusted meals are tried to validate his authentic insight, focusing his interest on ingredients that made up the food, cuisines and diet of these populations. Thus, he led the famous "Seven Countries Study" (performed in Finland, Holland, Italy, United States, Greece, Japan and Yugoslavia), so as to report the connection between lifestyles, nutrition and cardiovascular disorder between one of a kind populations, including through cross-sectional studies, being capable of prove scientifically the dietary price of the Mediterranean food plan and its contribution to the health of the populations that followed it.

From this research emerged an insight that clearly showed what the Mediterranean diet us capable of. This is because the populations that had adopted a weight loss program based totally on the Mediterranean Diet presented a totally low record of cholesterol within their people, and their blood was reported to be free from any disease. Consequently, a minimum percentage of coronary heart ailment was only recorded. This was so mainly because of the abundant use of olive oil, bread, pasta, veggies, herbs, garlic, red onions, and other ingredients of vegetable origin as compared to rather moderate use of meat.

The American nutritionist described the Mediterranean diet as the homemade minestrone, pasta of all varieties, with tomato sauce and a sprinkling of Parmesan, best sometimes enriched with a few portions of meat or served with a small fish of the region beans and macaron., a lot of bread, never removed from the oven a variety of hours before being eaten, and nothing with which spread it, plenty of clean maybe a couple of times a week and constantly clean fruit for dessert.

CHAPTER TWO: WHAT IS MEDITERRANEAN DIET PLAN?

If you're looking for a good and healthy diet plan which will help your vision, agility, body structure, weight and help increase your lifespan, then the Mediterranean diet might be just right for you.

The Mediterranean food plan blends the basics of wholesome consumption of cereal and grain with the conventional flavors and cooking methods of the Mediterranean.

Why the Mediterranean food plan and what is the Mediterranean diet plan?

Interest in the Mediterranean weight loss plan started out within the Nineteen Sixties with the commentary that coronary heart disease precipitated fewer deaths in Mediterranean countries, also with Greece and Italy, then in the U.S. and northern parts of Europe like Finland, Estonia, Denmark, Norway, Sweden, United Kingdom, Scotland, Wales and many other countries in that region. Many other relevant studies about food and their origins had observed that the Mediterranean food plan is associated with a reduced chance in heart problems and contains little or no elements and characteristics that are always responsible for a cardiovascular disorder, stroke and obesity.

The Mediterranean food plan is considered one of the wholesome and complete dietary plan or food plans advocated by many nutritionists, health practitioners and food scholars. Many of these nutritionists and health practitioners were able to research this dietary plan and eventually made available many workable and practical dietary guidelines for people all over the world. These guidelines have been known to help with fitness and save many individuals from continual sickness and diseases.

The Mediterranean dietary plan is also recognized and identified by the noble (W.H.O.)World Health Organization as a useful, healthy, perfect, cost-effective and sustainable dietary plan, formula or recipe and as a long-standing cultural asset by the United National Educational, Scientific and Cultural Organization which is simply known as UNESCO. This simply means that this food is not only cost-effective or useful for people leaving around Mediterranean areas or northern Europe, but it is as well useful, important and suitable for anyone who is looking for a way to improve their heart hygiene and improve their general wellbeing. Therefore, as you read on, I want you to prepare your mind for what you can harness from this book for your self-health and personal hygiene and fitness.

Mediterranean dietary plan, what does it mean?

The Mediterranean food plan is a way of eating primarily based on the conventional cuisine of countries bordering the Mediterranean Sea. While there's no sole definition of the Mediterranean eating diet, it is typically excessive in vegetables, lettuce, seafoods, complete grains, beans, nut and seeds, and olive oil.

The main components of Mediterranean weight loss program include:

- Daily intake of vegetables, fruits, complete grains, and healthy fats
- Weekly consumption of fish, rooster, beans, and eggs
- Moderate quantities of dairy products
- Limited intake of beef
- Other crucial elements of the Mediterranean food diet are sharing of food with family and friends, enjoying a glass of red wine and being physically active at all times.

Plant-based or vegetative meals, not meat-based, which means it is more of a vegetable than meat.

The foundation is being more of a vegan than not i.e. an individual becomes an herbivore by choice instead of being omnivores. What this portends is that the Mediterranean diet requires that you eat more vegetables and less of meat, low cholesterol, and carbohydrates. Mediterranean is simply more, roots, nuts, fruits, millet, carrots, herbs, nuts, beans, corns, legumes, water, a whole lot of grains and many more which I am going to discuss later in this book. Being the Mediterranean, it means your meals are likely to be built around those plant-primarily based recipes and your foods are likely to be like that of known vegans. Don't worry, you will get to eat your favorite chicken, fish and meat but at the minimum or lowest quantity not as you are used to. What I simply mean is that no matter how scared or desperate you are to get your Mediterranean diet off the ground, you can also get to include moderate and small quantities of dairy, turkey, chicken, meat, and eggs in your recipe and diet plan. This means that the mentioned types of non-plant-based foods and many more which I am going to discuss in the next chapters of this book also are crucial to the Mediterranean Diet. You get to eat seafood as you continue your Mediterranean diet journey. In contrast to the seafood which I will enjoin you to put more of it in your food, beef and any other types of red meat should be eaten only occasionally if you really want to stick to your Mediterranean food diet. It is necessary that you do that.

Healthy fat

Healthy fats and cholesterol are a mainstay and needed ingredients of the Mediterranean food recipe and plan. They're eaten instead of less healthful fats, along with saturated and trans-fat, which contribute to coronary heart ailment and cardiovascular disease. If you ensure that healthy fats and low cholesterol are duly observed in your diet plan, then you won't have to worry about heart failure.

Olive oil is the number one source of added fat in the Mediterranean food recipe or dietary plan. Olive oil gives mono or some types of unsaturated fats, which has been discovered to decrease overall cholesterol and low-density lipoprotein (LDL or "bad") ldl cholesterol levels. Seeds and nuts from the plants are also included in the class of mono or unsaturated fats and olive oil is one good oil to eat if you are looking for this type of oil in your diet.

Margarine or Butter

In the Mediterranean dietary plan, people always get confused about which one to eat, and what quantity to consume. They always look for validation on whether to consume butter or margarine. Margarine usually beats butter with regards to heart health. Margarine is crafted and processed from vegetable oils, so it carries no cholesterol, and it commonly has extra polyunsaturated and monounsaturated fats than butter does. But no longer all margarine is created equal or gives the same result, and some might also even be worse than butter. In general, the extra solid the margarine, the greater trans-fats it consists of. Look for a variety with the bottom calories that tastes in a good way on your taste bud, would not have trans fats and can be correctly said to have the very minimum amount of saturated fat that you can ever think of.

Fish are also critical to the Mediterranean eating recipe or dietary plan. Fatty fish — along with herring, mackerel, salmon, tuna, sardines, albacore, and lake trout — are wealthy in omega-3 fatty acids, a type of polyunsaturated fats that may lessen inflammation in the body. Omega-3 fatty acids also help lower triglycerides, reduce blood clotting, and decrease the hazard of stroke and coronary heart failure.

What about wine?

The Mediterranean food diet plan typically permits and gives some crimson-red wine in moderate quantity. Although in some quarters, alcohol has been identified to be a useful ingredient to some discounted threats of heart ailment in some studies, it is in no way to be claimed that I agree or disagree with their findings but I am using this medium to let you know that red wine has its own advantages and downsides and has been established to work and help treat some heart-related diseases. This means that even though if the red wine has its own downsides, it is useful if you want to implement this kind of Mediterranean diet plan that I am discussing with you in this book. For instance, in America, The Dietary Guidelines for Americans caution towards opting to drink or drinking more wine or alcohol frequently on the idea of capability health benefits of the red wine.

Why Is Nutrition from the Mediterranean Diet Important to Your Health?

Nutrition is important to live a healthy and long life, because what we eat matters. The food we put in the mouth is digested and used as nutrients for cell development and survival. Many people lack proper nutrition to nourish their body cells. Because cells lack adequate nutrition, a person can resort to overeating. Unfortunately, overfeeding does not lead to better nutrition. In general, incorrect substances are obtained, which negatively affect our level of health.

Eating well entails eating many fruits and vegetables since these food sources have the highest amount of nutrients. If you need to eat meat to get your daily protein intake, focus on lean meats such as fresh and salty fish and other poultry meat. Stay away from unhealthy meat like red meat.

In addition to eating well, you must fill your body with plenty of water, since H2O which is simply water in is one, if not the first nutrient that has the most vital nutrients which human beings need for their daily mental development and physical growth. It is one of the things that we cannot all do without on this planet. The human body is composed of 70 to 75 percent water and the human brain composed more than 95 percent water. Getting your body rehydrated is essential for your health and longevity.

STRESS REDUCTION: Stress reduction is important for a healthy lifestyle because too much stress leads to mental and physical illness and that is where this dietary plan coming. The Mediterranean diet plan is useful for stress reduction so if you are looking for a way to reduce your stress level this diet plan is the right way to go. Having a little stress in life is fine, but it should be balanced and eliminated whenever possible so since you have the option of eating Mediterranean, I beseech you to optimally use this plan for your stress reduction. Enduring too much stress for too long can make a person physically ill. Stress drains a person's energy, hinders cell communication, and forms nodes in the muscles of the body through tension.

Some forms of stress reduction include breathing, meditation, and exercise. Walking again is excellent for human health because it causes the body to move, pump blood, and reduce stress.

Eating the Mediterranean way

Are you really interested in trying out the Mediterranean diet for some months and would like to see how it is beneficial to your health and personal hygiene? These pointers below which I am going to discuss with you will help you get started on the right footing:

Eat greater culmination and vegetables. Aim for 7 to ten servings a day of fruit and vegetables.

Opt for complete grains. Switch to entire-grain bread, cereal and pasta. Experiment with other entire grains, together with bulgur and farro.

Use healthy fats. Try out olive oil in a large quantity and use it as a substitute for butter, and other types of oils and cholesterol infested oil or butter while cooking. furthermore, instead of choosing to put plenty of butter or margarine on your bread, ensure you start to dip your bread in the flavored olive oil in a manner that your bread is covered with flavored olive oil and is eaten like that. If you try this, you will start to see the difference in your look and your body in no time.

Eat greater and plenty of seafood in large quantities. Ensure you eat fish at least two times a week. Fresh fish or water-packed tuna, mackerel, salmon, trout, and herring are healthful choices that are useful for your health, especially your heart. Although grilled or smoked fish tastes in a way better and properly than canned fish and requires little cleanup, I still encourage you to eat fresh fish more. You must also try to avoid deep-fried fish at all costs as this is going to contain many things that you are running away from. Or do you think, it would be proper to eat fried-fish that contain more cholesterol than you can ever imagine? No, it is not proper so try to avoid such fish at all costs.

Reduce beef. Substitute fish, poultry or beans for meat. If you are a type that loves devouring meat always, ensure it is properly leaned and ensure such meat maintains small quantities of cholesterol. Beef should like to be eaten with utmost caution and should be eaten at a very low rate unlike fish

Enjoy a few dairy products. Eat low-fat Greek or plain yogurt and small amounts of a whole lot of cheeses every day. This will help to rejuvenate and give you the needed power and energy needed to function on your daily activities.

Spice it up. Ensure you always or usually include useful herbs and spices in your food. This will help to boost the flavor in your food and help to lessen the desire and need for salt in your food.

The Mediterranean diet is a scrumptious and healthful manner to eat. It is delicious and sumptuous, especially when eating with a purpose. Many of those people who get to switch to this style of eating say they will never consume any diet plan after trying it now. So, if you try it out after reading this book, you will be doing yourself a great service. But before then, let us look at other things as far as the Mediterranean diet is concerned.

CHAPTER THREE: COMMON MISTAKES AND MYTHS THAT SABOTAGE THE MEDITERRANEAN DIET

For many years now, researchers have studied plenty of diets and meal philosophies for distinct health advantages and benefits for human beings. When it involves overall gains, the Mediterranean food plan regularly comes out on top, supporting to reduce the danger of type 2 diabetes, heart ailment, and other persistent illnesses. The Mediterranean food plan refers to the traditional consuming styles of nations surrounding the Mediterranean Sea, including coastal elements of Spain, France, Italy, Greece, Turkey, Egypt, and Libya.

These areas generally tend to consume better quantities of fruits, veggies, whole grains, beans, nuts, seeds, fish, seafood, and healthy fat like olive oil—and lower quantities of crimson meat, processed foods, and delivered sugars. But adopting a Mediterranean food plan doesn't robotically make you healthier. As with any eating pattern, this heart-healthful food diet requires a piece of conscientiousness to avoid making blunders.

While your goal ought to in no way be perfection, and stability is essential, be cautious with these not unusual mistakes that would sabotage your Mediterranean diet:

1. Going overboard on oil

Yes, there's such an aspect as "taking an excessive amount of something good." While the Mediterranean weight loss plan is famous for embracing olive oil—and healthy fat in general—you may additionally want to keep away from freely dousing all your meals in swimming pools of oil. Think of it this way: The ideal quantity of fats is known to be the 30 percent of your total energy in a day, so you must aim for using simply one or two tablespoons in your meal on a day.

2. Going overboard on alcohol

One great aspect of the Mediterranean diet is wine, which simply means having a glass of wine with dinner—no longer than 1/2 a bottle is required by your body. It's true and right that alcohol has the useful ability and health benefits when consumed in small amounts, including a potentially positive effect on cholesterol levels, it can help burn unwanted cholesterol from the body. That said, the advantages that the alcohol gives to the human body can all be obtained from different yet less risky sources. This is because even though alcohol gives some benefits, it has a greater downside which weakens the human immune system, quick aging, can wreck kidney and damage liver if consumed in excess. Hence alcohol should be avoided at all cost and someone who is on the Mediterranean diet should source for the benefit that alcohol gives from different sources. Therefore vegetables are great source with which the benefits that alcohol gives human body can be derived without having to worry about its side effects on the body. In larger amounts, alcohol can carry critical risks, such as alcohol use disorder, hypertension, stroke, and breast cancer, in line with the American Heart Association. To stick with the Mediterranean food eating culture, make sure you add water in the right amount to most of your food recipes.

3. Speeding your food and rushing through your Mediterranean food is wrong

When doing the Mediterranean food plan, many people truly take proper cognizance of the food that is put on the plate and avoid any food that is not beneficial to their health, however, they sometimes rush through the food and fail to enjoy the food. This Mediterranean weight-reduction plan is a useful method for improving your life and a way of life or lifestyle that can enhance your lifespan. The Mediterranean weight-reduction plan emphasizes mindful, sluggish, and even pleasant dining. (Yes, a Mediterranean diet should no longer feel like deprivation or punishment; it should be enjoyable and must be enjoyed by an individual.)

Why must it be enjoyed? That's because consuming more slowly tends to result in more satisfaction from your meal, and studies have shown that people generally tend to ingest fewer calories while eating slowly. So, you must take advantage of that knowledge.

In other plain words, consuming while you are working or doing something as a pastime, even while working at your desk, or even as you are sitting in front of the TV may not be the right way to go about this. Instead, find a calm surrounding free from distraction, and consume your Mediterranean food in the company of other people when possible. To slow things down and lose some calories, always try so hard to ensure your spoons and forks being used to eat are put down in between bites. You can also do that by attempting to devour your food with chopsticks which the Chinese used for their food. Away from the mistakes and the myths, here are some useful guidelines that you could use to make a delicious Mediterranean diet.

The Mediterranean diet gets its fair share of (well-deserved) flack; however, concerning the clinical literature, there seems to be controversy over a Mediterranean-style weight loss plan which an individual can adopt. Rather than a rigid plan, the Mediterranean food plan is flexible and it is just like a mash-up of cuisines from the few countries that surround the Mediterranean Sea; however there are high percentage of a few features that different studies had shown which has to do with heart disease and Mediterranean dishes – it is believed that Mediterranean meals, heart-health and weight loss plan have some correlation and Mediterranean diet can help in treating heart diseases.

The Mediterranean food plan is known for plenty of colorful fruits and vegetables, fish and seafood, some grains, and fats like nuts and olive oil. It limits the intake of sugar and processed foods, saturated fats like red meats, dairy, and poultry products.

A 2013 study in European Journal of Cancer Prevention located proof that this aggregate of ingredients increased longevity in participants and reduced the risk of heart disease and certain cancers, and it may help save you and treat the type 2 diabetes, in keeping with 2014 take a look at Diabetes/Metabolism Research and Reviews. It can also enhance cognitive characteristics in older populations because of the monounsaturated fat, primarily based on a 2015 look at JAMA Internal Medicine.

Well, I know that many of us would instead want to increase the percentage of our baggage and move to Naples or Santorini, but the reality is it's perfect to add a bit Mediterranean flair to any meal, even those in everyday rotation on your own home menus. Here's how:

Flavor with herbs. Cooking with herbs like basil, cinnamon, coriander, oregano, and dill will let you cut back on the salt, sugar, and fats that commonly provide up in our food, in keeping with the American Diabetes Association. Another remarkable option? A cup of ora, like a squeeze of lemon juice or a bit orange zest.

Add sparkling vegetables to pizza. Here's how to make your pizza extra of healthy food. After baking, toss fresh arugula or toddler kale on top of your pie. Not handiest does it up the taste. However, it also adds a vibrant shade assessment in your regular red pie. Try it out: right here's an artichoke arugula pizza that you will neglect anything that will not be healthy or useful to your health.

Embrace the bean. Mediterranean recipes often consist of beans, which provide a healthy dose of fiber and protein. Add chickpeas or cannellini beans to your salad or in pasta. You may even add crunch on your salad via including roasted chickpeas.

Make half your plate roasted vegetables. Go-to veggies in the Mediterranean cuisine consist of eggplant, mushrooms, artichokes, potatoes, and tomatoes. (Fine, that ultimate one is technically a fruit, but it's still first-rate and good for roasting which can be combined with other cuisines.)

Make tzatziki your condiment of choice. This easy sauce is made from plain yogurt, diced cucumber, minced garlic, and sparkling herbs, like dill. Add it on your wraps and sandwiches, use it as a dip for carrot sticks, or maybe dress a Greek salad with it. Think of it as a more fit cousin to ranch dressing, and the opportunities are endless.

Add bean spreads to sandwiches. Whether you stick with classic hummus or venture into the opposite beans, this is a smooth manner to add flavor and protein to a sandwich. FYI, you could make a hummus-like spread out of almost any bean, so test with white beans, edamame, and some spice.
Try pine nuts. The Mediterranean weight loss program makes use of all styles of nuts, like walnuts and pistachios, but pine nuts are so smooth to add to savory dishes. They're right raw or toasted; simply toss them in your salads or in sauté vegetables.

Add seafood to pasta. Instead of including ground beef on your marinara or hen for your pesto, try shrimp, scallops, or mussels
Give new grains a chance. You've probably tried brown rice already; now supply lesser-regarded grains like bulgur, farro, or whole wheat couscous a shot. (Technically, couscous is a pasta

which I believe anyone would want in their diet, no longer a grain itself because of the process it has gone through.)

Prepare ingredients with olive oil. A word of caution: even though olive oil incorporates the precise-for-you monounsaturated fats, it's still oil that's great in calories and fat, so you want to consider how plenty you're eating at some point of the day. Also, extra virgin olive oil isn't supposed for high-warmness cooking, so transfer to avocado oil on your sauté needs.

Add eggplant—to everything. This versatile veggie soaks up anything taste you add it to, so it can move in honestly anything. Dice it up into one-inch cubes, sauté till soft, and mix it with portions of pasta, stews, and casseroles. You also can roast or grill in oblong slices and upload on your sandwiches.

CHAPTER FOUR: HEALTH AND MEDICAL BENEFITS OF A MEDITERRANEAN FOOD DIET

Daily pastime spent with others and sharing of food with others is vital factors, part and parcel of the Mediterranean Diet. These are sometimes important and needed if one wants to have a great Mediterranean diet and food. Spending time with others and sharing food with them can really have a profound effect on one's temper and intellectual or mental fitness. It can also help one foster a very deep recognition of the pleasures and reel the benefits of making healthful and tasty meals at the right time.

Of course, making modifications (whether losing or gaining) to your weight is rarely easy, especially if you're trying to stay away from the ease of processed and takeout ingredients. But the Mediterranean weight-reduction plan may be cheaper as nicely as a satisfying and very healthful manner to consume. Making the transfer from pepperoni and pasta to fish and avocados might also take a few efforts, however, you can soon be on a route to a more fit and longer life.

A traditional Mediterranean weight loss program consisting of massive portions of sparkling fruits and vegetables, nuts, fish and olive oil—coupled with physical interest—can reduce your chance of serious mental and bodily health issues through:

It prevents coronary heart sickness and strokes. Following a Mediterranean weight-reduction plan limits your consumption of delicate loaves of bread, processed ingredients, and pink meat, and encourages drinking pink wine in preference to tough liquor—all elements that can assist prevent coronary heart disorder and stroke.

It keeps you agile. If you're an older adult, the vitamins received with a Mediterranean food plan may lessen your chance of developing muscle weakness and different signs of frailty for about 70 percent.

It reduces the risk of Alzheimer's. Research indicates that the Mediterranean weight loss plan might also enhance cholesterol, blood sugar levels, and standard blood vessel health, which in turn may also reduce your chance of Alzheimer's sickness or dementia.

It halts and halves the chance of Parkinson's ailment. The high ranges of antioxidants in the Mediterranean food plan can prevent cells from undergoing a harmful process called oxidative pressure, thereby reducing the chance of Parkinson's sickness in half.

It also increases longevity. By lowering your chance of developing heart sickness or cancer with the Mediterranean food diet, you're reducing your risk of loss of life at any age through 20 percent.

Protecting against and help in treating type 2 blood sugar or diabetes. The right Mediterranean diet is rich in much fiber which can digest slowly, then work in a manner that prevents big swings in the blood sugar in the human system and will eventually let you keep a healthy and right weight.

Myths and records about the Mediterranean food plan
Following a Mediterranean weight loss plan has many blessings; however, there are still several misconceptions on exactly a way to take gain of the lifestyle to lead a more fit, longer life. The following are some myths and statistics about the Mediterranean food plan.

Myth 1: It feels very great to eat food this way.
Fact: If you're cooking meals out of lentils or beans as your primary supply of protein and choosing to stick with mostly plant-based fruit, vegetable, and much grains, then the Mediterranean diet is right for you. Instead of going for processed foods, opt for this type of diet.

Myth 2: Another myth is since a cup of wine is good on your coronary heart, then 3 glasses are 3 times as healthful for you than one.

Fact: Moderate quantities of pink wine (one drink a day for women; two for men) virtually has particular fitness blessings in your heart, but consuming an excessive amount of it has the opposite impact. Anything more than glasses of wine can certainly be bad in your coronary heart.

Myth 3: Eating massive bowls of pasta and bread is the Mediterranean way.

Fact: Typically, the Mediterranean people don't devour a large plate of pasta the way American people do. Instead, pasta is often an aspect of the dish with approximately a half cup to one cup added to their meal. The rest of their food consists mostly of salads, tuna, vegetables, beans, fish or a little portion of organic, herbivores meat, chicken, and perhaps one slice of bread which is made from fiber.

Myth 4: The Mediterranean weight-reduction plan is handiest about the food.

Fact: The food is a huge part of the food dietary plan. Yes, however, don't overlook the alternative approaches the Mediterranean also live their lives. The way the people from that part of the world contribute to their healthy living not just-food.

For instance, don't eat in a rush and they don't eat while watching TV. What they do is, they take a seat in a relaxed manner, leisurely eating their meal with others, which may be just as critical on your fitness as what's for your plate. The Mediterranean also enjoy lots of physical exercises and do activities that make them to burn unused energy or calories.

How to make the change

If you're feeling daunted with the aid of the notion of converting your eating habits to a Mediterranean diet, here are a few hints to get you started:

Eat plenty of vegetables for a long time. Try a simple plate of neatly diced tomatoes that are well drizzled with some olive oil and a bit of well-prepared feta cheeses. You can also stuff your thin pizza with many peppers and neatly prepared mushrooms as opposed to pepperoni and sausages that people regularly take. Salads, soups, and crudité platters are also outstanding approaches to load up on vegetables.

Always devour breakfast. Fruit, entire grains, and different fiber-rich meals are an awesome manner to begin your day, retaining you pleasantly full for hours.

Eat seafood twice a week. Fish together with tuna, salmon, herring, sablefish (black cod), and sardines are wealthy in Omega-three fatty acids and clams have similar benefits for brain and coronary heart health. You can also include some sort of shellfish such as mussels, oysters, periwinkle and/or crab.

To also have a good Mediterranean diet, try to cook a vegetarian meal at least one night a week. If it's helpful, you can bounce on the "Meatless Weekends" culture of leaving out meat, especially red meat, on the weekends in each week, or simply pick out a day where you build meals around beans, corns, and some vegetables. Once it becomes your habit, then you can add Mondays to your free meat days.

Intentionally choose dairy products in moderation. The USDA recommends limiting saturated fats to no greater than 10% of your everyday energy (approximately 200 calories for most adults). With this, you can continue enjoying dairy products such as natural (unprocessed) cheese, Greek or plain yogurt.

For dessert, consume sparkling fruit. Instead of ice cream, cake or different baked goods, opt for strawberries, fresh figs, grapes, or apples.
Use good fat. Virgin oil is best used, in fact, it is better to be a natural oil: nuts, olives, vegetables, sunflower seeds, and avocados are terrific sources of healthy fats in your daily food.

What to do about mercury in fish

Despite all the fitness blessings of seafood, nearly all fish and shellfish contain lines of pollutants, which include the toxic metal mercury. These guidelines can help you make the most secure choices.

The awareness of mercury and other pollution increases in larger fish, so it's pleasant to keep away from consuming massive fish like shark which has no tangible benefits, swordfish, tilefish, and king mackerel should also be avoided too.

The majority of the adults can safely eat about 12 ounces (6-ounce servings) of other styles of cooked seafood a week.

Pay attention to neighborhood seafood advisories to study if fish you've stuck is safe to consume.

For women who are pregnant with a child, nursing mothers, and children aged 12 and younger, select only plates of seafood such as shell fish o that are lower in mercury, such as shrimp, canned light tuna, salmon, Pollock, or catfish. Because of its higher mercury content, devour no more than 6 ounces (one average meal) of albacore tuna in keeping with week.

Make mealtimes a social experience

The simple act of speaking to a pal or loved over the dinner desk can play a massive function in relieving stress and boosting mood. Eating with others can also save you overeating, making it as healthy in your waistline as it's also for your outlook and other parts of your body. Switch off all electronic gadgets: TV, PDA, smartphone, your personal computers and join other members of your family over a meal. This is one way through which you can maximize the effects of your Mediterranean food on your body.

Always be in the circle of your relatives and stay updated with each other's daily lives. Share your heart and moods with them in order to be emotionally fit and happy. Having a regular dinner or lunch with relatives help you grow happy and good. This Mediterranean foods or diets offer consolation to little children, make them happy and are an awesome way to reveal their eating habits which can help you to know when they are about to get sick and when they are okay.

Share your Mediterranean food with other people in your community to expand your social circle and have a strong social network. If you stay alone, cook a little more and invite friends over to your house, Mediterranean food can be shared with a coworker, or neighbor and this is one way to enjoy your meal.

Cook with others. As I rightly invite you to share purchasing and cooking obligations for a Mediterranean meal. Choosing to have a Mediterranean food team-cooking with other members of your family or friends can be a very fun way to start and deepen a relationship between you and those people you choose to cook your Mediterranean food with. It can also be an unofficial method to share and split the charges and work. This could make it enjoyable for you and at the same time, cheaper.

Quick start to a Mediterranean eating habit

The easiest manner to make the trade to a Mediterranean diet is to begin with small steps. You can try this by:

- Sautéing meals in olive oil as opposed to butter.
- Eating extra end result and vegetables through enjoying salad as a starter or side dish, snacking on fruit, and adding greens to other dishes.
- Choosing entire grains as opposed to subtle pieces of bread, rice, and pasta.
- Substituting fish for crimson meat as a minimum twice in line with week.
- Limit high-fat dairy by way of switching to skim or 1% milk from 2% or entire milk.

CHAPTER FIVE: MEDITERRANEAN BREAKFAST

If you're following the Mediterranean weight loss plan, you realize you ought to be loading your plate with veggies and accurate-for-your proteins like salmon. But what about breakfast? Fruit, dairy, and entire grains play a large role in the weight-reduction plan, so there's actually a whole lot of tasty (and satiating) breakfast alternatives to select from. Here are 10 recipes to inspire you.

1. Caprese Avocado Toast

Avocado toast may not have originated in the Mediterranean, but its mixture of complete grains and wholesome fat makes it properly-suited to the food plan. This one feels more appropriate and better because of its Caprese salad twist which is good for Mediterranean breakfast.

2. Bacon-Avocado

This is the meal that is needed for strength and for looking radiant. It is a delicious recipe that you can prepare with 1 Avocado dissected into two equal half with the stone removed

To have this recipe you need 1 tablespoon of salted butter, 3 Large eggs, three slices of bacon cuts into smaller parts, a pinch of salt and a pinch of black pepper. This has to be mixed and cook for a while. See page 12 for cooking instruction...

3. THE CAULIFLOWER CARBONARA PAN MEAL

This is another sumptuous Mediterranean meal. To have this diet, you need 2.5 cups of frozen riced Cauliflower, eight slices of bacon, six finely chopped garlic cloves, 1 Tablespoon of dried Italian Herb seasoning, 1/2 tablespoon of salt, 1/2 cup of cashew cream (1/4 heavy cream and 1/4 cup of grated parmesan) and two yolks of egg. See chapter 12 for cooking instruction.

4. FLAXSEED CRACKERS

It is certain that after eating this meal for breakfast, you will want to have another great one the next day. This Mediterranean meal helps give you the strength when consumed in the right proportion. You will need 1 cup of flaxseed food, three tablespoons of olive oil, vinegar, 1/4 cup of apple cider, 1/2 tablespoon of water and 1/2 tablespoon of sea salt. See chapter 12 for comprehensive cooking instruction.

5. HEALTHFUL CHICKEN SALAD

Everyone needs the right amount of healthy fat to stay alive and be healthy. This Mediterranean meal gives you the required protein and fat that you need. To make this meal you must have in your possession, 2 cups of Chicken breast pieces, 2 cups of cut steamed green beans, 1/2 cup of homemade mayonnaise, 1/2 cup of diced pecans, 1/4 cup of diced cilantro, 1/4 cup of basil leaves, 1/4 cup of mint leaves, 1/2 tablespoon salt and 1/2 tablespoon of white pepper. See chapter 12 for detailed cooking instruction.

6. Eggs with Zucchini, Summer Tomatoes, and a sprinkle of Bell Peppers

To save the time which most people don't really have in the morning, you could decide to make, for your breakfast, the vegetable or plant-based food diet which you have cooked in the previous night can be warmed in a skillet for your breakfast. To fully enjoy this, you can add some eggs to it.

7. Poached Egg added to crisp White Beans or Green Bean

Although this breakfast recipe for Mediterranean diet calls for some sort of Swiss chard, any leafy green can also be used here. Therefore, don't think twice to use anything crisper in your kitchen for this breakfast.

8. Hazelnuts, Blueberries, and Lemon with Grain Salad for Mediterranean Breakfast

In case you have some simple or plain cooked quinoa that is leftover from dinner in the preceding night, use it for this wonderful breakfast. You can add to Hazelnuts, Blueberries & Lemon with Grain Salad to have a uniquely sweetened grains low carb salad that can serve as your breakfast when you are following the Mediterranean diet.

9. Chilled or refrigerated Wraps of Spinach Feta for Mediterranean Breakfast

I will enjoin you to make a double batch of these egg wraps. You can eat the first one at any time and put the second one in a freezer. the chilled wrap is what is good for your Mediterranean breakfast. This Spinach Feta is useful when you are in a hurry yet want to stick to your Mediterranean diet.

10. Avocado and Egg Breakfast Pizza

Opt for entire-wheat pizza dough to make this breakfast pizza more wholesome. You can also use complete-wheat grain, flour or different store-bought flatbreads to store time.

11. Spinach Artichoke Frittata for Mediterranean Breakfast

Marinated artichokes make sure this vegetable-packed frittata is full of flavor. Eat it heat or do like the Italians do: Enjoy it at room temperature or even cold.

12. Healthy Fruit Salad for Mediterranean Breakfast

Choose any mixture of fruits and entire grains to make this salad. You can eat any quantity and make it in your own way. You also can pinnacle a serving with a large spoonful of Greek yogurt to include a bit of protein in your diet.

13. Mediterranean Breakfast Pita

While those egg and hummus-crammed pita sandwiches are genuinely breakfast material, they'd additionally make a splendid packable lunch or easy dinner.

14. Easy Muesli for Breakfast

While muesli originated in Switzerland, its mix of complete grains, nuts, and fruit make it totally Mediterranean-friendly. Try pouring dairy or non-dairy milk over it or sprinkling it on yogurt.

15. Opt for whole-grain bread.

This easy and no-cook dinner meal can be cobbled together in moments and eaten at the go.

With entire-grain bread, you will be consuming greater fiber and nutrients than in white bread, and to help you stave off the ones mid-morning munchies. Peanut butter offers the ones high-quality, healthy fats with its protein, and the banana will upload some sweetness, greater fiber, and potassium.

16. English muffin with high nutritious toppings

Another smooth breakfast at the Mediterranean food plan is opting for an English muffin piled excessive with hearty toppings. Smear an entire-grain English muffin with bean spread earlier than adding a handful of potassium-packed spinach and a poached egg.

Any bean dip in oil will do here: hummus, black-bean dip, white-bean dip. It will pull the sandwich collectively right into a cohesive meal. With a bit salty and tangy flavor alongside its dietary punch, it is a wonderful stand-in for cheese, which should be used handiest sparingly.

17. Yogurt drizzle with a small honey

Greek yogurt is strained in a manner that makes it better in protein than ordinary yogurt. Yogurt is additionally wealthy in probiotics, which are exact bacteria essential for many physical functions. If you really want a bit of sweetness in your Mediterranean breakfast, you can upload a mild drizzle of honey. And, for a further crunch, attempt including ground flaxseed. It's rich in omega-three polyunsaturated fatty acids, which are extremely crucial for fighting inflammation in the body.

CHAPTER SIX: MEDITERRANEAN LUNCH

Making your Mediterranean lunch can be hectic, especially when you want to go the Mediterranean but if you follow these simple recipes which I am about to share with you, you will be able to save hundreds of cash which you would have spent on foods that are merely junk. Lunch is a perfect way to get on a fitness kick, and while consuming Mediterranean meals (also known as the full tomatoes, lemons, feta, or falafel you could place on one plate), you won't pass over those fatty subs one bit. You may find it difficult to go from your house to Greece and back when you want a quick taste of good food, but these delicious Mediterranean recipes that are both good for your body and that are definitely made for you.

1. Lemony Orzo Salad

This rice-formed pasta reigns in the known world of transportable and packaged meals. It is not perishable and brings energy. You've in all likelihood had your fair share on the menu being shared at summer picnics, so why no longer prep it for lunches all week? You can reduce the elements as you deem fit, but, if you can strive to include fresh carrot, neat cucumber, red or white onion, feta, many slices of apple, basil, chickpeas, mint, spinach, it would be so awesome.

2. Cauli Rice, And Chicken Cutlet

Cauli rice and cutlet is a lunch that you don't want to miss. It is both great for energy and at the same time protein and healthy vitamin that your body requires to function. To have this on your lunch menu, you need one small cauliflower, two tablespoon sesame oil, 1 Tablespoon coconut aminos, one egg, four tablespoon almond flour, 1 Tablespoon dashi powder, quarter of tablespoon salt and pepper, pinch of salt and pepper, one skinless bird/chicken breast, 40g beef rinds and frying oil (refined coconut oil) which is necessary if you want your lunch to be inviting. See chapter twelve for expressive cooking instruction.

3. Shirataki Noodles (Konjac)And Asian Salad

This is one of the popular menu on the Mediterranean diet. It is known as food which can help to stimulate brain and help one's vision. It is both and healthy and contain little fat. Tooo   hhhave this food in your Mediterranean menu, you need a Shirataki Noodles (konjac), two asparagus (40g), 1/2 cup of cucumber (65g), half of tomato (65g), one stem cilantro, one garlic, one egg, two tablespoons of coconut aminos, 1/16 red onions (20g), 1 Tablespoon fish sauce, 1 Tablespoon lemon juice, 1/2 tablespoon sesame oil, one-quarter of tablespoon salt and pepper and lastly, one-quarter of tablespoon of warm chili oil. To see how this can be easily cooked, check chapter twelve of this book for detailed instruction.

4. Falafel Kale Salad with Tahini Dressing

Homemade falafel, whenever I discuss it with people seems like a daunting task or recipe to make. In reality, you can make this Mediterranean lunch in just 10 minutes. To start, you'll be needing to blend together white onion, chickpeas and at least two garlic in a food processor or mixer. After that, you can then start to add cilantro, parsley, cumin, coriander, and red tomato and some pepper flakes. After you have successfully done frying up the falafel, your base salad is simply made: kale (marinated in lemon juice), red or white onion, white or green beans, and jalapeño.

5. Lettuce Meal

This is aother great homemade Mediterranean meal that one needs to have in his diet if he really want to maintain a youthful look. This meal requires two lettuce leaves, two chopped bacon, 8 tomatoes, half avocado, and tablespoon of mayonnaise, two lettuce leaves and on tablespoon of green peper. If you don't mind, you can add green beans but this is not necessary. For cooking instruction, see chapter twelve.

6. GRILLED COD AND SHRIMPS

People in the northern Europe are fond of this food which can be homemade and at the same high in nutrient that the body needs. What makes it a great source of right vitamin is the fact that its recipe is more of seafood than any other thing. It only requires two cod fillet, 1 tablespoon of lemon juice, two tablespoons of olive oil, two garlic cloves, eight cherry tomatoes, at least 200g shrimps, 2 stems fresh parsley, two garlic cloves. See chapter twelve for cooking instruction.

7. Gluten-Free Mediterranean Pasta

Nowadays there are so many alternatives to wheat and fiber. Therefore, wheat and gluten-free or fiber lover can simply have a portion of good Mediterranean food. This recipe makes use of brown rice noodles to go which can be added to roasted eggplant and some well sliced and prepared cherry tomatoes. Furthermore, there are other types that you would really like, and this includes chickpea- or quinoa-based pasta.

8. Classic Mediterranean Salad

A bowl of classic Greek salad doesn't really require anything to be added to it before you can have a good lunch—it's delicious enough on its own so there is no point adding another thing to it.

To start you can prepare some spinach, cherry tomatoes, black olives, with thinly diced onion (the red one), and you can also add your beloved cheese (mind you this has to be a salty one), and there must be little feta in it. For an easy dressing to healthy, combine olive oil, purple wine vinegar, minced garlic, Italian seasoning, salt, and pepper.

9. Mediterranean Lentil Salad

Lentils are a pantry object that can virtually keep as much as anything—stews, soups, you call it. This recipe has them starring on their very own with the assist of purple onion, radishes, celery, red bell pepper, parsley, and feta. What is the quality part of this recipe? You could have a big batch prepared in less than 30 minutes, and it'll maintain for days.

10. Greek Turkey Meatball Gyro with Tzatziki

You do not just want a Greek giagiá for a meal at any time of the day, I bet you want if for your lunch. having it for lunch is the best way to go. Instead of the regular lamb which can be used as your meat (we all know this is too pricy and would cost you a fortune, therefore you must find an alternative), you should rather go for this meal. Having this for lunch will make you look younger and fight aging. This recipe can stand as a replacement for your tasty turkey meatballs. You can even prepare it by wrapping it in a pita and top it with tzatziki. Try this and you won't want to have another thing for lunch. Well, the fact is, anything (meal or meat) covered inside or with a cucumber yogurt sauce is far better for your health.

11. A bowl of Mediterranean Pepper Sauce that is well roasted With Quinoa

No more sloppy, saggy or watery salad lunch for you as this is the best thing to replace your salad with. A great bowl of quinoa, that is stuffed with cucumbers, some Kalamata olives, feta cheese, onion (the red one), hummus, mantil, basil, and a dollop of fried red pepper sauce is the best Mediterranean diet that you need for your lunch. You should prepare this with caution.

12. Greek Shrimp Souvlaki and Farro Bowl

This is a lunch that you don't want to miss in your weekly lunch. A plate of this should include herb mixed with shrimp, red peppers, some lemon and a handful of zucchini, tomatoes, and olives. All those mentioned items for you to make your food a great one. This Mediterranean recipe requires full-grain farro, but you could use quinoa or even brown rice, and this is so good for those who are interested in gluten-free food.

13. Greek Lemon Chicken Soup

This soup plays flawlessly with avgolemono sauce (egg and lemon), which, if you've tried it, is probably in your top-foods list, like ever. The reheat value on it is wonderful too (so ideal for the workplace microwave).

14. Lemon Parmesan Chicken with Zucchini Noodles

We always love our zoodles complete of garlic and lemon—the cheese is simply a bonus ingredient. All you want to be prepared to do is meal-prep is butter and dried oregano (that you in all likelihood already have), chicken, garlic, lemons, a broth of your choice, and lots of Parmesan.

15. Quinoa Stuffed Eggplant with Tahini Sauce

This full-grown, stuffed, and thick eggplants are easy lunch for your Mediterranean lunch. I will enjoin you to load your belly with the whole thing that goes into this great recipe: quinoa, garlic, mushrooms, sliced plum tomatoes, carrot, onion, and self-made tahini… You'll have a rethink on why you should eat salad bar instead of this great Mediterranean eggplant.

16. Bulgar Salad with Feta

Bulgar can without problems keep its personal as the principle dish to your lunchbox. This one is greater lemony and pairs perfectly with all of the first-class herbs: cilantro, mint, and parsley. As for the must-have topping, you've got feta, that's first marinated in lemon zest, garlic powder, and fresh oregano. Hello, salad of our dreams.

17. Mediterranean Veggie Sandwich

When all your preferred toppings grow to be the principal event, you realize lunchtime will be good. This sandwich, which is largely a salad between two slices of complete-wheat bread, has lettuce, sprouts, tomato, crumbled feta salted cheese, cucumber, red pepper, white onion, and for its star: peppadew peppers (both candy and spicy are useful in this recipe). If you are thinking about spreads which you should add, try any hummus. However, you should realize that this recipe requires that you eat as lunch and not as dinner.

Top Mediterranean Dinner Recipes & Entrees

1. Greek-Style Baked Cod with Lemon and Garlic

There is a cause this baked cod recipe has been the first choice of cooked and enjoyed recipe of many people in the Norway, Sweden and Estonia! A handful of Mediterranean spices, plus a combination of lemon juice, olive oil, and garlic, give it glorious flavors! This food plan can be put together in just over 20 min or less. It is a good source for needed nutrients and can be used to suppress diabetes.

2. Arugula Salad With Basil Vinaigrette

Many people who are keen on losing unnecessary weight always find this meal helpful. In fact, some people who are into keto use this Mediterranean recipe just to get a fast and accurate result for their Keto plan. This food is better taken as dinner because it is light and useful for faster result. To have this meal, you need 40g arugula, five to six slices of cucumber, three tomatoes, two slices prosciutto, three broccoli florets and 1 serving basil and

Vinaigrette. For cooking instruction, check the chapter twelve of this book.

3. BROCCOLI AND ROSEMARY CHICKEN

I will advise you take this serious as it can help you feel good. This meal is useful for people who are young and looking for ways to avoid quick aging. It requires one boneless bird leg, one-quarter tablespoon of salt, half of tablespoon of rosemary, 1 tablespoon of olive oil, one-third of broccoli, 1/4 tablespoon of black pepper and small quantity of water. Please see chapter twelve for cooking instruction.

4. Kale Beef and Vegetables Wrapped In Avocado and Olive Oil

This is number choice for the old people who are trying to maintain their youthful look and sharp brain. This Mediterranean meal is also good for the treatment of high blood pressure. For a plate and one person meal of this diet, what is required is half of avocado, two tomatoes that are evenly sliced, one portion of Caesar dressing, one massive kale leaf, 1/8 purple onion, 100g thinly sliced beef, one quarter of tablespoon of pepper, salt, and garlic powder, 1 tablespoon of olive oil. See chapter twelve for the cooking instruction.

5. Mushroom and Broccoli and Bacon Meal

For a vegetarian who is looking for Mediterranean alternative as dinner, this one is more decent and proper for you to have. To have this, you must have 8og of broccoli, four big but brown mushrooms, at least three portions of bacon, one-quarter of tablespoon of salt, half tablespoon of rosemary, one-quarter of tablespoon of garlic powder and a pinch of black pepper. See chapter twelve for comprehensive cooking instruction.

6. Garlic and Lemon with Greek-Style Baked Cod

Garlic and Lemon with Greek-Style Baked Cod Mediterranean Recipe. this recipe can be cook with baked bread, carrot, garlic and some fresh lemon juice which is needed for a healthy body. While cooking this dinner, you should also endeavor to add olive oil and garlic to the menu. This Mediterranean dinner should not take more than 15 mins or 20 for it to be prepared so you can make this when you are so hungry. See chapter twelve for cooking insstruction

7. Chicken Shawarma

This crisp yet pristine Mediterranean baked bird shawarma is what is common in the Middle East and it is a good meal for a dinner! It has many great tastes that for the health of both your eyes and heart. The crux and flavor in this meal are in the simple homemade shawarma spice mixture that you are cooking. I bet after eating this dinner, you will be so happy with yourself.

Homemade Chicken Shawarma fresh fowl shawarma recipe is good for your dinner! With sprinkled spices, and olive oil made from marinate. This recipe can be eaten with salad, vegetable etc.

This flavored and colorful shawarma is one dinner that you must include your dinner Mediterranean routine.

8. Moroccan Vegetable Tagine

A simple self-made vegetable stew stuffed with warm Mediterranean Dish is good for your health. An easy and succulent vegetable stew, flavored Moroccan-style with warm spices, aromatics, and dried apricots are all that you should consider in your dinner. The satisfactory vegetable tagine or vegetable stew should be combined with fruits and vegetables.

9. Easy Seafood Paella

A contemporary and clean version of seafood paella with shrimp and lobster. You'll love this rice dish. And no unique paella pan needed! Step-by-step educational and video blanketed with the recipe.

Seafood paella in a cast iron skillet

10. Spanakopita

Savory Greek pie manufactured from flawlessly flaky phyllo dough with heated spinach and feta cheese filling. It's less difficult to make than the maximum people think. Check out the recipe and tutorial.

Spanakopita Recipe (Greek Spinach Pie) high-quality recipe, for a way to make spanakopita: Greek spinach pie with crispy, feta cheese, golden phyllo and a smooth filling of spinach, and herbs are required for your Mediterranean dinner.

11. Chicken Souvlaki

The right to home-made hen souvlaki is within the marinade! It's so easy to make, but the correct stability of flavors.

This home-made chook souvlaki recipe is what is popular in Athens. therefore, you should consider it in your Mediterranean dinner. This food is not complete without the high-quality souvlaki marinade; This recipe is good for both indoor dinner or outside dinner and can be served together with some grill and wine.

12. Briam

If you're looking for a vegan principal or a hearty side, Greek Briam will now not disappoint you and will make a great dinner. This recipe is similar to the ratatouilles, Briam can be said to be a combination of stunning vegetable, although it is more flavored than it and actually good for your dinner when baked and made crispy. Briam. zucchini, with Regular Greek roasted Vegetables, red peppers with potatoes, onions (the red one), tomatoes and additional virgin olive oil

13. Grilled Kofta Kebabs

Skewers of floor beef and lamb blended with fresh parsley, onions, garlic and heat Middle Eastern spices.

Top Mediterranean Recipe of 2016 fragrant fowl lemon soup, organized Greek-fashion. If you've had it at your nearby Greek restaurant, you know how comforting this bird rice soup is. And this homemade model is so good for your health and it is very easy to prepare at home. If you really want a great Mediterranean dinner, this is the right one for you. A related recipe is Greek avgolemono soup and I enjoin you to try this out.

14. Italian Baked Chicken

Boneless skinless chicken breasts organized with an easy spice mixture, garlic and extra virgin olive oil, and finished with clean parsley and basil. Italian Baked Chicken with Tomatoes. Garnished with Basil and Parsley

15. Moroccan Lamb Stew

Comforting dinner, as this is good for your dinner if you want to maintain your Mediterranean diet. Soft braised lamb is what is most required in this recipe, chickpeas, white onion, warm Moroccan flavors and some green pepper are what are required in this recipe.

Moroccan Lamb Stew with Vegetables for dinner is one good way to end your day so you should use this if you are eating out or having a family dinner in your home.

16. Falafel

If you've ever wanted to strive homemade falafel from scratch, my message in this book is all you need to get it done! You can follow the simple recipe that follows. Hearty and wholesome vegan patties made of floor chickpeas, garlic, and sparkling herbs. This is as real as the actual falafel recipe vendors and eatery serve people who are looking for a Mediterranean diet. Falafel wraps with fresh vegetables and tahini sauce.

17. Shakshuka

Turn a few eggs into the precise meal with this simple shakshuka recipe! Eggs poached in a flawlessly-spiced vegetarian stew of tomatoes and green peppers. Perfect for breakfast, lunch, or even The Mediterranean Dish. Shakshuka is a scrumptious Middle Eastern dish of eggs poached in a spiced, saucy tomato stew. Perfect for breakfast, lunch or dinner! All you want to add is your favored bread. This is a simple vegetarian recipe that you may make in less than 30 mins! My family's favorite. And with that, you can feed dinner to a handful of people on a small budget.

CHAPTER EIGHT: MEDITERRANEAN DESSERT

Since you've determined to commit to the Mediterranean recipe and diet, you're in all likelihood now not going to consume dessert every day, however, you have to live and you need dessert after your food sometimes. And to me and people around, let me tell you, living a good life means eating the sweet stuff not occasionally but when you feel like. If you have for once sunk your enamel right into a forkful of lemon cake or a fudgy brownie, then you will realize what's up and what dessert can do to your daily living. To provide you with something to look forward to, I have compiled those Mediterranean desserts that are good for your body and can be followed. These desserts or recipes, food plan can also be used by anyone who is trying to diet or lose weight without going against any rules of good diet at all.

For this recipe, you will need to change butter for olive oil and you must also put whole-wheat flour in your dessert as opposed to refined flour. These Mediterranean dessert treats deserve a front-and-center spot in your next dessert, so come along with me as I reel or you realize, some personal interest to create some useful dessert for you:

1. Italian Apple Olive Oil Cake

For individuals who like their desserts no longer so lip-puckeringly sweet, this cake can be your new go-to dessert as it is the best choice for those people looking for the right dessert after their meal. Don't be afraid that you might some weight, eating this dessert will lead to no such thing— I can categorically tell you that you're doing it in the right way. Also, this isn't always the time to scrimp out and get reasonably-priced greater virgin olive oil; go for the right oil if you want to have a great dessert.

2. Low Carb Bread

Many people prefer this as a dinner but I am telling you that you can have this as dessert as well. What is required to have a great dessert from this is four tablespoons of easily grounded almond meal, one-quarter of tablespoon of baking soda, one huge egg, two tablespoons of water, three tablespoons of olive oil, and one-third of tablespoon of salt. Check chapter twelve for comprehensive cooking instruction.

3. THE MEDITERRANEAN ALMOND BUTTER BURGER

This dessert helps you to gain stamina and helps to treat forgetfulness or partial amnesia. Two tablespoons of grounded turkey, two tablespoon of apple cider, one vinegar, one large egg, half cup of almond butter crunchy and unsweetened, two ground tablespoon of black pepper, 1 tablespoon of fish sauce, one and half of tablespoon of turmeric, a half of tablespoon of garlic salt. See chapter twelve for explanation on how to make this dessert.

4. ASPARAGUS, SAUCE AND AVOCADO BOAT MEAL

This is one of the favorites of the people who want to recover quick from sickness. It is a good dessert to have in order to look fit and healthier. The main ingredients for this include asparagus, sausage and avocado boat. Furthermore, 60g sausage, 1 or 2 asparagus, 1 Tablespoon olive oil, one or half slice of an avocado, 70g tuna, one-quarter cup of dry spinach, one tablespoon of mayonnaise and lastly, green pepper and, a pinch of vitamin A salt are what are needed. Please check chapter twelve for a detailed explanation on how to make this dessert.

5. SESAME SALAD AND CHICKEN BROCHETTES

I love having this one for dessert. With it, your dessert can never go wrong as it contains what is needed by the body to have a radiant skin and great bone. To prepare this dessert, three chook, vegetable brochettes, three lettuce leaves, one tomato slice, one portion of sesame dressing, one quarter of avocado are all needed. Preparing this dessert doesn't require a special expertise. See chapter twelve for a detailed direction on how to cook it.

6. Popped Quinoa Crunch Bar

This is the right dessert for adults and young children who are trying to stick to the Mediterranean diet. While the look of fatty food is great, the popped quinoa in this self-made dessert which can bring some critical crunch and crisp dessert to your table. Take one-quarter cup of a very dry quinoa that has been fully heated in a very heavy-bottomed pot, and I assure you that it will remodel itself from its uncooked grainy self to something nutty, crisp, crunchy and tasty. Trust me on this, you'll need popped quinoa as part of your desserts more often than not.

7. Honey Almond Ricotta Spread with Peaches

When you're in the temper to indulge in something extra savory and cheese-filled for dessert instead of the plain cookies, this is the dessert that is crunchy yet crispy, it is a cupcake that is delicious and at the same time creamy. This recipe is just too good for your dessert and should always be included in your dessert. To have it good and tasty, you should sweeten it with a hint of nuts, honey, and fruit, grape, carrot and this spread is excellently served with a toasted slice of whole-grain or wheat bread.

8. Blueberry Muffins for dessert

One key a part of the Mediterranean diet is kicking butter to the slash and swapping in olive oil. This recipe does simply that, and it also calls for adding a few whole-wheat doughs into the mixture of what you have, which gives it a nuttier, heartier taste. Have I mentioned that you may whip up this dessert and its ingredient less than 10 minutes?

9. Flourless Chocolate Olive Oil Cake

This chocolate olive cake dessert might look like it should be left to the professional's cake-makers or caterers to make, but no you too can make it at home and use it as part of your dessert. Try to imagine this dessert as a huge fudge brownie that everybody can make with an introduced hint of espresso flavor. Don't skimp at the satisfactory and make certain to bake it with chocolate that contains at least 70-percentage cocoa.

10. Healthy Energy Bites

These electricity bites are just as true for a pre-exercise snack as they're some kind of dessert with your family and friends, a dessert that is both cheap and sweet, then this is for you. Also, if you are really looking for a dessert that you can have any time, you definitely will understand this is the necessary dessert that you require in your life. The self-made recipe is packed with simple and healthy elements like dried apricots, cashews, shredded coconut, dates, and citrus zest. Gluten-free, Paleo, and vegan eaters alike must all bookmark this recipe ASAP.

11. Roasted Fruit

You felt like you were given bad news when you are told to eat roasted fruits, right? Caramelizing isn't most effective for red onions. In a case that you are a fan of fruit and vegetables but looking for something a bit greater satisfying than biting right into a raw apple, then you should attempt roasting your favorite fruits inside the oven with brown sugar. This recipe calls for the handiest five minutes of preparation and four ingredients: clean blueberries, cinnamon, peaches, and some brown sugar. We wager apples and pears might taste pretty darn excellent too.

12. Whole Grain Citrus and Olive Oil Muffins

These muffins feel as much as they look. They are prepared from flour, carrots, almonds, rolled oats, and white onions, orange, which can be later studded and decorated with chopped almonds on it. To sweeten this dessert, you will need some lemon juice, orange zest, maple syrup, you will also definitely need orange juice, and vanilla extract. This is how your dessert for breakfast can be made by yourself.

13. Vegan Lemon Olive Oil Cake

In a case that you get to know that your relatives or friends are coming over in an hour time without informing you prior the time you get a call, this is the type of dessert that you really need to impress them, this lemon cake is a quick one to get creative and place a great dessert on your table for your friends. However, I need to warn you that you'll be whisking some not so usual ingredients like lemon or orange juice, brown sugar, olive oil, milk, not-sweetened almond milk, some lemon zest, and whole-wheat pastry dough. The fine element is the fancy candy glaze on top that is somehow most effective in this dessert. You also need some powdered sugar, some vanilla extract that you can find and lemon juice.

14. Pistachio No-Bake Snack Bars

When you want a bit kick but can't drink any other cup of coffee, this pistachio snack bar is the precise energizing mixture of nutty and candy. In your shopping cart, you'll need: pitted dates, pistachios, rolled old fashioned oats, pistachio butter (use almond if that's what you have got on hand), unsweetened applesauce, and vanilla extract. Be prepared to combat during the last bite.

15. Maple Vanilla Baked Pears

Thanks to this easy dessert, we now understand that we in reality like our fruits manner higher whilst they may be dripping with maple syrup. You will be throwing together pears (preferably Mediterranean pears and I believe you have the idea of this pear), pure maple syrup, cinnamon, and pure vanilla extract. Dessert's up in 25 mins.

16. Olive Oil Chocolate Chip Cookies

Everyone desires a reliable chocolate chip cookie recipe for themselves and to have their pocket free from spending too much money. Prove your baking prowess with those olive oil-crammed sweet treats with a view to have your pals accomplishing for seconds (in case you don't get to them first). Swap out the semisweet chocolate chips for darkish chocolate chunks or shavings that have more than 70-percentage cocoa. I am sure many people likely have the rest of the components of the ingredients needed for this dessert in their kitchen. Therefore, this is a simple Mediterranean dessert that you can make for your people or yourself at any time of the day.

17. Fig Almond Olive Oil Cake

You don't even need to be a daughter or son of the richest man to have the recipe of this dessert on your table. In fact, you can get it right at first try if you can follow my suggestion. First of all, I will like you to see this much like a pound or mashed cake. However, one thing I want you to consider is that it is much less dense with its almond flour and olive oil filling. You'll recognize it's ready

when the edges and your sweet fig look brown and reach some
ideal or natural color.

As handy as packaged snacks are, homemade ones not only flavored better, crispy, crunchy and good but are also cheap and easy to make than those at the stores. This means they are easy to make and can be incredibly easy to make by anybody who wants Mediterranean snacks. The following Mediterranean snack recipes can deliver not only delicious but good fat and snacks and will not make you the vending machine or snack that you can get in stores.

1. Mediterranean Thin Crust Flatbread

I know you are currently asking about the major difference between a pizza lunch and a flavored flatbread snack, right? For starters, this recipe is going to be solely heavy and laced with the veggie toppings and should be very low on the crust and cheese, which means you're getting more of those nutrients and much less of the ingredients that can make you have post-pizza bloat. But do to fret or think you will not be able to have a good snack: Less cheese doesn't mean much less taste, right? If you believe so then you do not have anything to be scared about. If you choose to still use burrata way to make your Mediterranean snacks, the creamy level is still so excellently high so no cause for alarm in any way. I will enjoin you to use your dinner or lunch leftover for this snack.

Instead of wasting your leftover, you can turn them to the Mediterranean thin-crust flatbread snack. Simple!

2. CHICKEN GRILLED THIGH WITH ZUCCHINI SALAD

Personally, I enjoy this snack as it is yummy and at the same time healthy for someone who is trying to take up Mediterranean diet. This requires one-quarter of zucchini, 1/4 purple pepper, five basil leaves, one garlic clove, one fowl thigh with a skin of (75g), 50g Swiss chard, half of tablespoon of salt and pepper, 1 Tablespoon of olive oil, 1 tablespoon of vinegar, three tomatoes at least. See chapter twelve for a detailed analysis on how to make this snack.

3. GRILLED SALMON AND GREEN BEANS AND RADISHES

For anyone looking for a great snack after a long hard day and strenuous work, this one is for you. It is better if it is served hot and made at home. For it to be perfectly made 150g of salmon fillet is needed, three tablespoon of olive oil, half of tablespoon of salt, two tablespoon of black pepper, dill, 1 tablespoon of lemon juice, 1 tablespoon of rosemary, five radishes, pinch of salt, garlic powder, and pepper, one garlic clove, and 80gram of green beans (and carrots) are needed. See chapter twelve for further instruction on how to prepare this snack.

4. MEDITERRANEAN BAKED OMELET

I can bet it that you will definitely love this snack as it is devoid of red meat, anything that can make you add more calories but has more of wheat flour. To make this snack what is mostly required is browned and crumbled sausage, wheat flour, 10 great big eggs, with a cup of nice whipping cream, you can also add one cup of ground Cheddar cheese, half of tablespoon of salt, green pepper, dill, chili, and other seasonings, to make your Mediterranean omelet sweet and well flavored. See chapter twelve to understand how to effectively cook this snack.

5. Smoked Salmon Goat Cheese Endive Bites

Are you still unsure about what to do with the leftover of your Mediterranean lox? I will advise you to pack up those smoked salmon, add a few endive leaves to it, then spread the well-preserved goat cheese on it for the last low-carb. After that, add some wholesome-fats to your afternoon snack. Even though the endive leaves are quite sturdy, I advise leaving the spreading on it. You can also prepare it ahead of the time that you think you might need some snacks this is because you can have it handy if it is prepared before it is needed. Furthermore, after being topped with freshly chopped or diced dill in order to have a few herby freshness, and to preserve its flavor, I will advise you coat it with garlic, herb, fine goat cheese, white onion, and black pepper (all these are needed for this snack to taste better).

6. 15-Minute Mediterranean Chickpea Salad

Salads can genuinely make terrific snacks—in particular, while they're full of protein, like this easy chickpea blend. However, because you don't have lettuce in your kitchen does not stop you from having a great snack so no need to fear about snacks becoming soggy or having mold overnight. In fact, I will advise you making a huge batch of this Mediterranean snack on the weekend—the longer it stays and gets soaked inside the dressing, the flavored it becomes. With that, you can choose to pack it in a dish and put it into a single-serve bin and choose to take with you whenever you're on the move. For this snack to have greater protein, you can decide to add diced chook or salmon, or mackerel or canned tuna.

7. Loaded Mediterranean Hummus

Hummus alone is a very delicious and super snack. But loaded hummus is absolutely the type of snack you want to have. You can choose to top it with crunchy cucumber, spiced chickpeas, onions, juicy tomato, creamy feta and lots of clean herbs. If you still want to stick to your Mediterranean snack, then this is the most useful recipe to keep in your fridge and bring out whenever hunger strikes. Use whole-wheat feta, and pita chips or crackers for the Mediterranean food plan.

8.   Crock-Pot Chunky Monkey Paleo Trail Mix

I am sure you are now wondering about what you can do with crock-pot. Well, I am going to tell you what to do. For a great Mediterranean snack, you need cashews, coconut flakes, carrot, walnuts, and Paleo-pleasant chocolate which must be well tossed into the pot (with coconut oil and vanilla extract included and well blended with it). Therefore, to make a crock-pot chunky monkey paleo Mediterranean snack you must make a dessert-like snack that won't come up with a high sugar or snack that is high in carbohydrate and saturated fat.

9.   Smoky Loaded Eggplant Dip

Yes, I am still going to talk about hummus because it is needed for most snacks. I know everybody is always up for trying some new things and they want to do it differently. Whether you are currently feeling chickpea fatigue, or you are desiring to change your snacks and spicing things up, I will advise you always to have this eggplant handy and always have it within reach for your next snack. Smoky, loaded yet stiffed with more vegetables (cucumber, carrot, watermelon, green pepper, white onion and tomato can be best used to top your eggplant dip Mediterranean snack). You can also sprinkle it with toasted pine nuts if you don't mind. Let me tell you a fact, this dip is the exceptional snack you need while you're craving a feeling that has to do with eating something creamy. It's additionally a superb filler for the popular feta and pita and it is a useful snack just like the Mediterranean quesadilla.

10. Peanut Butter Banana Greek Yogurt Bowl

Everybody knows that granola, carrot and the Greek yogurt are so delicious (and very clean). Well let me ask you, have you ever tried yogurt with melted peanut butter as a snack in your life? Let me inform you: It's a sport and life-changer, you only need to try it out as you have now decided to try out Mediterranean snack. Vanilla Greek yogurt is in addition flavored with a sprinkle of nutmeg and crowned with honey and sliced or diced banana, peanut drizzles and ground flaxseed for the healthier snack that also tastes great and good. For some hearty and healthy grains in your snack, ensure you add unsweetened granola, honey, and feel free to add whatever sparkling fruit you have got on hand.

11. Mediterranean Roasted Chickpeas

Trade-in your chips snacks for this great, salty, sweet and flavored roasted chickpea. To have it as the very best snack, you should spice it with oregano, and black pepper, garlic, onion, green pepper, wrap in dill and doused in lemon juice, carrot, and purple wine vinegar. As you continue to eat this great snack, those crunchy bites get better every day in your fridge. To avoid over-snacking (they're that so good to be used as snack), put the snack into a well-packed container whenever you are traveling, and you believe you will need a great snack for yourself. This Mediterranean snack can be eaten both at home and outside. They also taste excellent when sprinkled with some fruit salads or vegetable salad or combined with homemade veggie chips which are also another nutritious element that should be included in your diet.

12. Savory Feta Spinach and Sweet Red Pepper Muffins

Savory desserts are simply worth savoring every time. Full of feta, basil, spinach, margarine, paprika, and green peppers, these egg-filled desserts are a superb single-serve snack to have handy any time of the day. Change the whole-wheat flour to maintain it consistently with the Mediterranean diet and you should also feel free to experiment with it. You can choose to do that by adding other veggies, like a mushroom, broccoli, okra or sun-dried tomato at any time.

13. Baked Whole-Grain Lavash Chips and Mediterranean Dip

Why buy pita chips while you can make your very own with two simple substances? Though these are technically lavash chips, the flavor just like pita but are a hint thinner—which means you may eat that many greater, right? You can choose to dip into the lemon parsley dip if you like. You can do that by making some recipes from scratch or opt for store-sold chips. After all, it is possible that you probably already made the chips.

14. 7-Ingredient Quinoa Granola

Granola is high-quality, but now and again we need something with a little extra protein. When we don't want to rely totally on Greek yogurt for that boost, we turn to quinoa. Left raw so it can become extremely good crispy, this quinoa-filled granola makes for a super bowl of cereal, quick snack (sans any more elements), or, of course, topper for yogurt. Throw in sparkling or dried berries to lift it up that rather more and feel loose to bypass the sugar.

15. Greek Yogurt Spinach Artichoke Dip

Who stated spinach and artichoke dip isn't healthy?! Whoever did, in reality, hadn't met this recipe. Yes, it has cheese (3 to be exact), however it without a doubt receives a majority of its creaminess from Greek yogurt—a Mediterranean food diet favorite. Using an entire percent of frozen spinach, this dip delivers just as a lot on the greens as it does in gooey goodness. It even tastes first-rate with veggie dippers, like carrots and bell peppers, so you can load up. (Do it for the veggies.)

16. Smoked Salmon, Avocado, and Cucumber Bites

Cucumber bites aren't just a fantastic party snack, and they're also a first-rate snack in general. Full of healthful fats from smoked salmon and avocado and crunch from the cucumber, these bite-size eats are an appropriate technique to snacks when you're searching to maintain matters low-carb. In case you cannot get avocado, then you should probably look for pears to add to this recipe. This is the right snack for those who are so keen on the Mediterranean snack.

17. Whole-Wheat Banana Blueberry Muffins

These whole-wheat, banana and blueberry truffles would make us nothing but to feel great and happy. Full of fiber, carrot, banana, honey oats and whole-wheat flour and some different taste from the nutmeg, maple syrup, blueberries, and butter. Well, those truffles are a great on-the-cross snack or comforting chunk which you need to have handy whenever you are feeling the pang of hunger.

I believe this snack can be eaten by anybody irrespective of their diet choice and food plan.

CHAPTER TEN: VEGAN ALTERNATIVES

Trendy dietary plans like ketogenic and others are the quick skirt-sporting cheer captains in this scenario, even as the Mediterranean food plan is virtually carrying t-shirts and sitting within the bleachers. It's been here all along, and (that is wherein my Swift analogy ends) it comes with a laundry listing of science-sponsored benefits. So, despite the fact that it's no longer usually at the top of thoughts, the Mediterranean weight-reduction plan will, in no way, go out of style as it has been in existence for so many ages and would always be sought after for its benefits and medicinal values.

Being a vegan can sometimes make it tough to put into effect a new pattern of eating into your life and start a new life — after all, if you've managed to figure out the protein and omega-three resources that work for you in a way, why would you then choose to mess with it? But if you are a vegetarian, it might be really worth giving the Mediterranean recipe or diet a try.

This is so because, as a vegan, probabilities are pretty is so high that you already eat most of the foods considered a part of the Mediterranean food plan.

It's definitely an easy weight loss program to observe in case you are vegetarian or vegan. One thing you should realize is that this diet is based on a foundation of whole grains, leaves, greens, and some fruit. Where it is distinctive then [the typical meal or everyone diet is known to include meat, poultry, and fish. These are handled so much as greater and more important kinds of a dish than a major dish.

Here are the satisfactory meals to eat in case you're a vegan trying to attempt the Mediterranean recipe. When I think of a standard meal on the Med eating diet, I imagine much like, a ton of salmon. So, following a Mediterranean-fashion ethos while you're also vegan may not seem especially intuitive. But lo! It genuinely makes a ton of sense. "The Mediterranean food plan is a superb plan to observe in case you're vegan given that the weight-reduction plan focuses mostly on plants, whole grains, fruits, and veggies anyway," That's because the famous consuming plan is "greater of a way of life than a diet, just like being vegan is," she says. "It's all approximately enjoying your meals, listening to your hunger and fullness cues, and consuming loads of domestically sourced wholesome ingredients."

That stated, there are some things you should hold in thoughts when trying to integrate the two ingesting plans. Here, Berman breaks down how to effectively follow a vegan Mediterranean weight loss plan.

1. Prioritize omega-three fatty acids

Omega-three fatty acids, which can be found in some types of fish and oils are an important part of any wholesome eating plan;

they're fantastic in your brain, and this recipe can also enhance the physical appearance, look, glow and health of your individual skin. This vitamin if used at the right proportion can also help you slow down aging. These are the needed ingredients that the vegans can also use as they try to eat Mediterranean diet: Fish is known to be one of the richest sources of these fatty acids so as a vegan you might want to avoid it and go for, are glaringly great vegetables off the table.

Thankfully, you continue to can get enough of those vital fatty acids if you devour the right meals. "There are 3 main varieties of omega-3s: ALA, EPA, and DHA. ALA is mostly found in plants, and EPA and DHA are determined in fish," Berman explains. Your body converts ALAs to DHAs (the gold trendy of omega-3 fatty acids) but it's now not a particularly green process. While Berman notes that maximum human beings consume approximately one to 2 grams of ALA per day, "ALA isn't as well-absorbed as the type that comes from animal resources," she says, meaning vegans might want to consume greater. But research result is varied on the exact amount that is useful so would consult with your health practitioner before trying out a particular amount.

Many food experts recommend that an individual who wants to stick to the Mediterranean diet should strictly adhere to consuming meals like flaxseed, chia, walnuts, and tofu to hit your even quota. Plus, many experts note that Mediterranean meals are also proper sources of protein.

2. Be clever about your diet and take the right amount of protein intake

The Med weight loss program isn't restrictive, like a few different plans (cough keto cough), and there are plenty of vegan alternatives that fit in the plan's framework. "Definitely make certain you're ingesting protein and omega-three sources at each meal to stay glad and get the vitamins you need," Berman says. That can come from beans, entire grains like quinoa, nuts, seeds, and different vegetarian protein ingredients. (Check out this listing of vegetarian meat options for more ideas.) "In addition, vegans need calcium from resources like green, leafy veggies, sesame seeds, and tahini."

"As with any vegan diet, you also want to make certain you're getting enough of nutrition B12, which isn't found in plants," Berman adds. You can do that thru fortified cereal, a food expert once says, or let me say a food expert once recommends speaking to your physician to know and identify the first option and technique that can work out for you.

3. Go for variety

"A well-rounded Mediterranean plate has protein, fat, and fiber," Berman says. "Breakfast will be savory oatmeal or other whole grain with nuts or maybe hummus, whole wheat pita, and veggies." Lunch could appear like a bean salad with olive oil, parsley, and couscous, even as dinner will be something like tofu, spinach, and quinoa with fresh fruit for dessert.

Beans are a first rate and go-to food to get protein, fiber, and prevent heart disease, according to the American Heart Association. They are also an important issue of the Mediterranean weight loss plan.

"Beans, being a type of food with so much protein, are so commonly eating in the Mediterranean, yet right here it's almost an underrated superfood. They seem to be ubiquitous in many of our supermarkets, but many just do not like eating them due to the fact they don't know what to exactly do with them and they do not know what they can actually use them to make apart from cooking as a food.

To get your legume restored, try washing, perhaps soaking for sometimes, then blending some beans, for instance, kidney beans, chickpeas, or black beans, or lentils, or it can even be cowpeas. Blend this with some sort of salad, soup, onion or platter of sautéed vegetables. Just make certain you do rinse them because this is a great way to minimize and limit the consumption of sodium.

Tofu is a good meat replacement choice.

Mapo tofu.

You must have tofu a couple of instances a week. Gontabunta/Shutterstock

The Mediterranean weight loss program relies much less on meat than a few different diets.

Even fish and poultry, which ought to be eaten at the least twice a week, within the Mediterranean diet, are frequently handled as greater of a "unique occurrence" than a popular component of a meal, in line with food professionals and experts.

To ensure you're getting enough protein, attempt adding small quantities of tofu (which is manufactured from soybeans, making it Mediterranean weight loss plan-friendly) to your food a few instances a week.

Nuts and seeds provide you with the omega-three you need. Mixed nuts

Nuts can update the omega-three fatty acids that human beings now and again get in fish. Shutterstock

If you do not eat fish, it is able to be hard to get omega-3 fatty acids. As a replacement, I will advise including nuts and seeds which include chia seeds, walnuts, cashew nut, hemp seeds, and high quantity of flaxseeds. It is certain that all of those nuts offer protein as well as omega-3s acid which is really required by our body system to grow.

That stated, plant-based totally assets of omega-3 include a sort of omega-three that is much less active inside the body than the sort that comes from animal resources, in line with Healthline. Because of this, you'll want to devour a number of plant-primarily based omega-3s or upload a supplement to your food diet.

Whole grains upload extra fiber to your weight loss plan.
Quinoa stuffing
Another thing that is necessary for the who are looking for an alternative for a vegetarian alternative is that trying to eat whole grains, wheat is more nutritious, delicious than the white flour in our diet.

It is even better to switch from white flour content to whole grains as that will help your heart and brain. Some of the whole grain that you can eat are quinoa, corn, sprouted bread, and complete-wheat bread and pasta. This will, in a great measure, add fiber to your weight-reduction plan and help you live fuller and purposeful life for a longer quantity of time - this means that it contributes to longevity and a good lifespan for people who choose to eat this type of diet.

Vegetables are an essential part of the Mediterranean weight loss plan.
red onion, ginger or bell pepper are also useful.

Any vegetable is a useful recipe that you can also include in your diet.

One issue that absolutely everyone on the Mediterranean weight loss plan ought can successfully use as a staple is vegetables. Any form of vegetable you choose is fine, but you can't go wrong with dietary powerhouses which you may also discover that many people go to different Greek restaurants to eat. This includes recipes such as white onions, red peppers (bell one), mantil, broccoli, cabbage, spinach and carrot.

Fruit is a superb manner to satisfy your sweet tooth.

Blackberries

Blackberries are excessive in antioxidants and vitamins. Dwight Because the Mediterranean eating diet limits brought sugar, many nutritionists and health practitioners recommend getting your sweet and preservatives extracted from the fruit. Try ones excessive in antioxidants and vitamins, like grapefruit, blackberries, oranges, and raspberries.

Oils like olive oil can be multi-purpose.

Olive oil

Olive oil and canola oil are precise to prepare dinner with. The Mediterranean eating diet also emphasizes oils, like olive and canola oil. Try the use of extra-virgin olive oil to prepare dinner with or as an awesome salad (cabbage, carrot, spinach which is dressed or dipped in olive oil.

Mediterranean diet should be taken as a complete lifestyle, not just an eating plan.

Mediterranean Diet healthful meals tomatoes

The Mediterranean diet may be sustained as a way of life change.

Whether you are a vegan or not, it is highly essential to consider the Mediterranean food plan. I will enjoin you to give a second thought now and see the differences it can make in your life. I believe it is useful for losing weight and as well, it is a way to look fitter and healthier. However, the greater good of this diet plan is the fact that it is a great plan to enhance one's fitness, youthful look, save, money and overall to have a fine and peaceful life.

CHAPTER ELEVEN:
MEDITERRANEAN FOODS, EXERCISE, NUTRITION AND THEIR CONTRIBUTION TO LONGEVITY AND EXCITING LIFESPAN

Longevity is defined as a term that commonly refers to "long life" or "enormous duration of life." The word "longevity" is sometimes used as a synonym for "life expectancy" in demography. There are ways through which the Mediterranean diet contributes to long life and extends one's lifespan. This chapter will look at how exercise, nutrition and the Mediterranean diet can greatly help the human lifespan and ensure longevity in human beings. Several factors contribute to the longevity of an individual. Even among those who do not desire eternal life, one could desire the longevity of experiencing more than life or making a greater contribution to humanity. It can help make medicine for longevity and a longer and healthier life a reality.

Current research on aging and longevity shows that life expectancy is now 74 and 80 years and could be significantly longer with the anti-aging advances that are currently being investigated. This research suggests a promising way to find and develop medications to prolong life and prevent or treat aging-related diseases. These ideas could shed light on human aging since it is known that humans and some bacteria have mutually beneficial relationships. The idea behind the dividend on longevity was clearly expressed in a book by the scientist that claimed that the research should have had the direct objective of delaying the seven-year aging process. The researchers were also interested in the influence of healthy and less healthy foods on mortality.

1. The Basic of Longevity

The secrets of longevity are the basis for living a healthy and harmonious lifestyle and existence. With degenerative diseases so rampant in our societies with cancer and cardiovascular diseases at the top of the list, it is necessary to return to the basics. Creating a fundamental basis for achieving and maintaining a healthy existence should be our first objective.

To achieve this basic basis, we must continually focus our attention on certain areas that shape our physical, mental, and emotional development. Three important aspects that require our attention are nutrition, exercise, and stress reduction. When we can master these three areas of self-development, we can live a longer and healthier life.

NUTRITION: Nutrition is important to live a healthy and long life, because what we eat matters. The food we put in the mouth is digested and used as nutrients for cell development and survival. Many people lack proper nutrition to nourish their body cells. Because cells lack adequate nutrition, a person can resort to overeating. Unfortunately, overfeeding does not lead to better nutrition. In general, incorrect substances are obtained, which negatively affect our level of health.

Eating well consists of eating many fruits and vegetables since these food sources have the highest amount of nutrients. If you need to eat meat to get your daily protein intake, focus on lean meats such as fresh and salty fish and other poultry meat. Stay away from unhealthy meat like red meat.

In addition to eating well, you must fill your body with plenty of water, since H2O is one of the most vital nutrients on the planet. The human body is composed of 70 to 75 percent water and the human brain composed more than 95 percent water. Getting your body rehydrated is essential for your health and longevity.

The exercise is important since the human body was designed by God, Nature or the Universe to move. The movement is part of our existence. To do anything, we must have a realm of uninhibited and unlocked movement. However, when we do not get the exercise that the body requires to remain flexible and agile, it oxidizes. The body does not need intense exercise to get a good workout.

Walking is an excellent form of exercise. If you walk during the day for 20-30 minutes, you can exercise daily and the vital nutrients that sunlight provides to humans. Other forms of exercise that keep the body full of energy and vitality include yoga, qigong, tai chi, and Pilates. For yoga and Pilates, you should focus on delicate styles that tone your muscles and test your level of flexibility and strength.

STRESS REDUCTION: Observing the Mediterranean diet plan, comes with its own stress, so how do you reduce your life stress and other unnecessary stress which can affect your health in the long run? Stress reduction is important for a healthy lifestyle because too much stress leads to mental and physical illness. Having a little stress in life is fine, but it should be balanced and eliminated whenever possible. Enduring too much stress for too long can make a person physically ill. Stress drains a person's energy, hinders cell communication, and forms nodes in the muscles of the body through tension.

Some forms of stress reduction include breathing, meditation, and exercise. Walking again is excellent for human health because it causes the body to move, pump blood, and reduce stress.

If you can concentrate on these three basic lifestyle options (nutrition, exercise, and Mediterranean foods), you can establish a longevity basis for yourself.

2. The Best Exercise Routine for Longevity When You Are Observing Mediterranean Diet

Walk fast for an hour every day.

It doesn't have to happen suddenly. For instance, if the train station is a 15-minute walk from your home and you do it anyway, it's 30 minutes there. Therefore, you can choose a cafeteria 15 minutes' walk from your office and make a daily visit. These may not be your exact circumstances, but an idea is made: find places that can be explored on foot and go there every day. On weekends, ensure you walk everywhere you go, even in faraway places: do your best to leave your car in the garage or at the entrance of your home throughout the weekend.

Cardiovascular exercise for 2.5 to 5 hours per week.

Running, biking or swimming are good options, but the type of exercise you choose is not important. The key is to work your body to the point of breathing quickly and sweating. A simple way to reach this threshold is to have a stationary bike and a road bike (to leave when the weather permits, otherwise go home) and take a 30 to 40-minute walk every two days and a total of 2 hours at the end of the week

This may be the classic routine in the gym, but your muscles get stronger when you climb the stairs instead of the elevator (Longo advises you to climb the stairs always!), Walk instead of driving, grow food in your garden instead of buying them, and do manual work at home instead you choosing to hire someone to do it. When participating in a weight training session, consume at least 30 grams of protein in a single meal within 1-2 hours to maximize muscle growth.

In terms of weekly runtime, research shows that most of the beneficial effects are caused by the first 2.5 hours. For example, a study conducted in Australia which had more than 200,000 respondents, aged 45 to 75 found that those who exercised (at moderate or vigorous levels) at least 2.5 hours a week had a 47% reduction in overall mortality. The increase of 5 hours per week led to a 54% reduction in mortality. Ensuring that at least part of this activity is in the vigorous range has reduced the risk of death by 12 percentage.

Another extensive study involving more than 650,000 people in the United States and Europe has shown that mortality has been reduced by 31% for people who have practiced at least 2.5 hours a week with moderate intensity (or more than 75 minutes at vigorous intensity). The increase in total exercise at 5 hours at moderate intensity (or 2.5 hours at vigorous levels) reduced the risk of death by 37%.

Examples of physical activity you can practice include walking fast or jogging slowly (faster than 4 mph), biking (10-12 mph) or gardening. Examples of strenuous physical activity involve climbing stairs or walking, cycling (more than 12 mph), playing soccer or jogging (more than 4 mph).

Therefore, there is undoubtedly an additional benefit of going up to 4 hours of training a week, with some of the exercises and training. There might be diminishing returns after 2.5 hours and you want to avoid overloading your body by going beyond the weekly limit of 5 hours. Excessive exercise causes damage to the knees, hips and joints over time. You do not want your body to break prematurely due to excessive exercises.

3. Energy Production

A key ingredient for longevity is energy and this can be found in the Mediterranean food plan. Energy feeds all organ systems, including the heart and the brain. Body energy production and how its production can be fully maximized will be discussed at this point.

The primary source of all biochemical energy comes from nutrients. The nutrients in food are decomposed or broken down by metabolism from higher to a lower energy level. As a result, energy is accumulated for personal use. Without energy we cannot move our bodies, nor would we be able to think correctly and create thoughts.

What type of nutrients provides the body with optimal energy? The science behind longevity is interested in advanced nutrient selection. However, high energy metabolism also depends on the logical use of the numerous cofactors that are relevant to the dynamics of metabolism: enzymes, minerals, vitamins and, where appropriate, nutrients derived from botanical substances and new molecules discovered through new medical research and analysis.

The body energy production depends on the adequate functioning of mitochondria, and the subcellular organelles specialized in the extraction of energy from nutrients. All that the body needs are well available in the Mediterranean diet and therefore it is certain that that type of diet plan can greatly contribute to long or short lifestyle of an individual depending on their due observation of this Mediterranean diet plan. Cell types differ in their mitochondrial content. For example, the heart, which needs constant vigour, has cells that contain several thousand mitochondria each; Skin cells, on the other hand, can function with a few dozen. Brain cells are also energy-intensive. Each organ has specific types of mitochondrial populations with unique and different requirements. Longevity training implements the new science of biological energy to expand the life span and quality of life.

Effects of Mediterranean Diet and Food Plans on Human Mind and Body

As the body strengthens, the mind also strengthens, and this forces the mind to master new patterns of experience that conserve energy and activate health.

Through special techniques adapted individually, the mind is trained to create special states of consciousness that give vitality to the networks of the body.

What experiences are sought in these special states of consciousness? Although each person may report differently, a comforting sense of tranquillity, a relaxing experience of detachment and a greater perception of physical strength and personal power are often expressed. Many people often admit that they experience pleasant feelings, have a peaceful state of mind and become happy when they are at home. Words often do not adequately describe these special states.

The neural basis of the power of mental images: The images, as used in longevity training, involve the conscious creation of mental representations that may contain visual images such as scenarios of dreams, sounds, words and phrases that are rhythmically pleasing and, above all, pleasant feelings and primary emotions.

Mental images derive from consciously activated brain areas. Neurons from different parts of the brain are well represented in the images used, each corresponding to extensive neural networks. The more diverse the images, the greater the areas of the brain that act and the more effective the therapeutic impact is when the waves of the neural networks resonate at the edges of the nervous system.

Healing images in longevity training must be individually adapted to respect the preferences of conscious and unconscious minds. Each practice reinforces healing images, expanding its systemic reach, working on reprogramming the neural substrate of the mind permanently.

4. Pro and Cons of Mediterranean Diet When Not Done in Proper Proportion

Following the Mediterranean weight loss plan may additionally result in greater stable blood sugar, lower cholesterol and triglycerides, and a lower risk for heart disease and other health problems.

How to Follow the Diet

The Mediterranean weight loss plan is based totally on:

Plant-primarily based meals, with simply small amounts of lean meat and chicken

More servings of complete grains, fresh end result and vegetables, nuts, and legumes

Foods that certainly contain high quantities of fiber

Plenty of fish and other seafood

Olive oil as the main supply of fats for making ready food. Olive oil is a healthy, monounsaturated fat

Foods that are eaten in small quantities or not at all among the Mediterranean diet plans include the following:

Red meats

Sweets and other desserts

Eggs

Butter

Possible Health Concerns

There can be fitness concerns with this ingesting fashion for a few people, including:

You may begin to gain some weight at some point in time if care is not taken. This might come as a result of consuming fats in olive oil and nuts.

You might also have decreased levels of iron. If you pick out to observe the Mediterranean diet, make sure to eat a few foods rich in iron or in vitamin C, which facilitates your frame to absorb iron. You may have calcium loss from ingesting fewer dairy products. Ask your fitness care provider in case you must take a calcium supplement.

Wine is a common a part of a Mediterranean ingesting fashion however a few people have to no longer drink alcohol. Avoid wine in case you are susceptible to alcohol abuse, pregnant, at danger for breast cancer, or have other conditions that alcohol should make worse.

CHAPTER TWELVE: A WEEKLY PLAN OF MEDITERRANEAN DIET

This is a four-week roaster that is designed for weekly Mediterranean recipe for those who want the best out the Mediterranean diet.

1. First Week

The Mediterranean food plan is a high fats, low carbohydrates, and good enough protein eating diet that is used essentially to treat difficult to control epilepsy in children. It is also useful in burning frame fat and dropping weight.

The following Mediterranean eating diet recipes are made with clean and perfect components that are wholesome for the body and can be gotten from grocery shops close to you. The food includes cooking instructions that can be effortlessly understood as you put together your recipes.

The following are a number of the Mediterranean diet recipes that will help you successfully gain your goals:

BREAKFAST

DAY 1	AVOCADO MEAL
	INGREDIENTS FOR AVOCADO MEAL
	1 Avocado dissected into identical 1/2 with the stone removed
	1 Tablespoon of salted butter

	3 Large eggs
	Three slices of bacon cuts into smaller parts
	A pinch of salt
	A pinch of black pepper
	COOKING INSTRUCTIONS
	1. Spoon out maximum of the avocado flesh leaving about half inch across the avocado
	2. On a low warmness, area a frying pan then, upload butter. While the butter is melting destroy the egg into a bowl and beat them adding the black pepper and a pinch of salt
	3. Add the bacon to one quit of the pan and permit them to fry for a couple of minutes without stirring. Then, upload the eggs at the opposite bottom of the pan and blend as they scramble. Within five mins the eggs and bacon ought to be equipped, however if the eggs get completed before the bacon you can dispose of the eggs and location it in a bowl
	four. Then blend the bacon portions and egg in a bowl and scoop it into the avocado bowl, and the meal is ready to be eaten.
DAY 2	THE CAULIFLOWER CARBONARA PAN MEAL
	INGREDIENTS FOR THE CAULIFLOWER CARBONARA PAN MEAL

i. 2.5 cups of frozen riced Cauliflower

ii. Eight slices of bacon

iii. Six finely chopped garlic cloves

iv. 1 Tablespoon of dried Italian Herb seasoning

v. 1 / 2 tablespoon of salt

vi. 1 / 2 cup of cashew cream (1/4 heavy cream and 1/4 cup of grated parmesan)

vii. Two yolks of egg

COOKING INSTRUCTIONS

1. Heat a massive frying pan on average warmness

2. Ensure to use a very sharp knife to cut the bacon into slices. When the frying pan is warm, add the bacon into the frying pan

four. Cook by using every so often stirring till the bacon is in the main crispy for approximately 6 mins

five. Add the finely chopped garlic

6. Stir thoroughly till the garlic begins to show brown

7. Add within the cauliflower rice then salt and dried herbs

8. Stir thoroughly until the rice begins to soften out, and any liquid produced evaporates.

9. Add the cashew creamer, this is the heavy cream, and while it is added you can start to prepare dinner with this creamer. You can then stir till it thickens, well-formed, and creamy. Then you can serve hot to

	your people.
	10. Top the serving with the clean yolk of an egg and blend in. The warmth of the cauliflower will cook dinner the uncooked egg yolk
DAY 3	FLAXSEED CRACKERS INGREDIENTS FOR FLAXSEED CRACKERS i. 1 cup of flaxseed food ii. Three tablespoons of olive oil iii. Vinegar iv. one-quarter cup of apple cider v. half of tablespoon of water vi. half of tablespoon of sea salt COOKING INSTRUCTIONS 1. Get a Container and mix all the ingredients. Mix till properly-shaped then go away it for 20minutes 2. Preheat the oven on 320F convection bake 3. Using a Turner to transfer the flaxseed blend to a sheet of bakery paper then cover with another foil and make it flat four. You can make use of a rolling pin to make it greater flatten till a square shape is shaped, then dispose of the top sheet of the bakery paper and pass the foil at

	the bottom with the dough on it to a baking pan then pop within the oven and bake within 40-45 mins until the middle is firm. That is when you tab it, it needs to be solid 5. Place it away from the oven and permit it cool to room temperature, then switch the bakery paper with cracker mass to a slicing board and with a big kitchen knife reduce into squares to make your preferred shape.
DAY 4	HEALTHFUL CHICKEN SALAD INGREDIENTS FOR HEALTHFUL CHICKEN SALAD i. 2 cups of Chicken breast portions ii. 2 cups of reduced steamed fresh beans iii. 1/2 cup of self-made mayonnaise iv. 1/2 cup of diced pecans v. one-quarter cup of diced cilantro vi. 1/4 cup of basil leaves vii. 1/4 cup of mint leaves viii. half tablespoon salt ix. 1/2 tablespoon of white pepper COOKING INSTRUCTIONS 1. Cut and dice your herb, pecans and green beans then portions the chicken 2. In a big bowl placed all the elements and mix gently

	to mix it up 3. Ready to eat
DAY 5	MEDITERRANEAN POKE MIXED WITH AHI TUNA AND CITRUS INGREDIENTS FOR MEDITERRANEAN POKE MIXED WITH AHI TUNA AND CITRUS i. 8oz Yellow Fin Ahi Tuna fillet ii. 1 Tablespoon of coconut aminos iii. Five sprigs cilantro iv. 1 / 2 Haas avocado v. Two tablespoons of sesame seeds vi. 1/4 cup of pili nuts vii. 1 Tablespoon of sea salt viii. 1 / 4 ruby red grapefruit COOKING INSTRUCTIONS 1. Cut your Ahi Tuna into one-quarter-inch cubes and places right into a big bowl 2. Next, add for your coconut aminos, salt, and sesame oil. Mix gently 3, Halve your grapefruit, cuts into exclusive sections then upload them on your bowl 4. Finely chop your cilantro and encompass it right into a bowl 5. Dice your pili nuts, chop your avocado, add it to the

	bowl and lightly mix to mix the ingredients 6. Divide the Ahi Tuna mix between bowls and decorate with sesame seeds.
DAY 6	TOMATO SALAD, BACON AND EGG INGREDIENTS FOR TOMATO SALAD, BACON AND EGG i. Three slices of bacon ii. one-quarter purple pepper iii. 1/4 Zucchini iv. Two eggs v. Pinch of pepper and salt vi. Three slices of tomatoes vii. One basil leaf viii. 1 Tablespoon of olive oil ix. 1 / 2 tablespoon vinegar x. One garlic clove xi. Sprinkle pepper COOKING INSTRUCTIONS 1. Slice the zucchini and crimson pepper 2. Fry the bacon in a small nonstick frying pan till it turns crispy. Place the bacon on a plate. Fry the zucchini and peppers within the bacon fat until it's tender. Sprinkle the pepper and salt over. Put at the

	plate with the bacon. three. Finely chop the garlic clove and basil leaf. Mix the olive oil, vinegar, basil, garlic, salt, and pepper in a bowl. Add the tomato chopped to the plate and pour the dressing over.
DAY 7	ZOODLES AND AVOCADO CREAM MEAL INGREDIENTS FOR ZOODLES AND AVOCADO CREAM MEAL i. One zucchini ii. half of avocado iii. 20 basil leaves iv. Three brown mushrooms v. 1/5 tablespoon of olive oil vi. One garlic clove vii. 1 Tablespoon of lemon juice viii. 1/4 tablespoon of salt COOKING INSTRUCTIONS 1. Cut your zucchini in a spiral shape. 2. Slice the mushrooms into halves. three. In a stick blender cup, mix the avocado, basil leaves, 1 tablespoon of olive oil, garlic, salt, and lemon juice. Press the on button at the stick blender for approximately 1 minute to permit the combination of the substances for a remarkable creamy and yummy.

	4. Add half of the tablespoon of olive oil in a saucepan and prepare dinner the mushrooms until it is smooth, then upload the zucchini noodles and prepare dinner for 1 minute or more until it gets warm. 5. Add the avocado cream and mix the entirety, then serve.

LUNCH

DAY 1	CAULI RICE AND CHICKEN CUTLET INGREDIENTS FOR CAULI RICE AND CHICKEN CUTLET i. One small cauliflower ii. Two tablespoon sesame oil iii. 1 Tablespoon coconut aminos iv. One egg v. Four tablespoon almond flour vi. 1 Tablespoon dashi powder vii. one-quarter tablespoon salt and pepper viii. Pinch of salt and pepper ix. One skinless bird breast x. 40g beef rinds

	xi. Frying oil (refined coconut oil)
	COOKING INSTRUCTIONS
	1. Dice the riced cauliflower in a part of meals via the use of a cheese grater. In a neat saucepan that you have put on stove, heat the same oil and put the riced cauliflower. Fry for about ten minutes, then start to add the coconut aminos, dashi powder, salt, and pepper then blend properly. Fry till the cauliflower is crunchy and smooth
	2. Grind the pork rinds using a meals processor or your palms. Mix the beef rinds with pepper, salt, and almond flour. Break the egg in a bowl, upload it to different elements and whisk the whole thing.3. Chop the fowl breast in 2 lengthways. Sprinkle the pepper and salt on both sides and dip into the whisked egg. Coat the hen with the breading on each quit.
	4. Fry the cutlet in temperature of 150C / 300F preheated oil and fry until the internal temperature of the bird cutlet is 65C /150F. You can serve with the cauli rice.
DAY 2	SHIRATAKI NOODLES AND ASIAN SALAD
	INGREDIENTS FOR SHIRATAKI NOODLES AND ASIAN SALAD

i. Shirataki Noodles (konjac)

ii. Two asparagus (40g)

iii. 1/2 cup of cucumber (65g)

iv. half of tomato (65g)

v. One stem cilantro

vi. One garlic

vii. One egg

viii. Two tablespoons of coconut aminos

ix. 1/16 red onions (20g)

x. 1 Tablespoon fish sauce

xi. 1 Tablespoon lemon juice

xii. 1 / 2 tablespoon sesame oil

xiii. 1/4 tablespoon of salt and pepper

xiv. 1/4 tablespoon of warm chili oil

COOKING INSTRUCTIONS

1. Place some water in a pot to boil. Put the egg in the water and simmer for 7 minutes exactly. Once cooked, do away with the egg and put it in a bowl of ice water. Peel the egg and cut it into four pieces.

2. Wash the shirataki noodles underwater and boil for two minutes. That will really get rid of the smell. In the same pot consist of the asparagus and prepare dinner till tender. Drain the water and allow the noodles and asparagus to settle down. You can smash the noodles into smaller parts.

	three. Dice the purple onion with a cabbage shredder then reduce the asparagus into 1/2. Chop the tomato, slice the cucumber, cube the cilantro, and finely chop the garlic the use of a garlic crusher. 4. Pour all of the ingredients, at the same time, right into a bowl, then integrate properly. Ensure to serve bloodless.
DAY 3	LETTUCE MEAL INGREDIENT FOR LETTUCE MEAL i. Two lettuce leaves ii. Two chopped bacon iii. 1/4 tomato iv. half avocado v. 1 Tablespoon of mayonnaise vi. Two lettuce leaves COOKING INSTRUCTIONS 1. Ensure you start cooking by frying the bacon in a neat and good saucepan until it turns crispy and inviting. 2. Chop the tomato into a few slices, chop the avocado as nicely. three. Use half of tablespoon of mayonnaise over every lettuce leaf and cover with the bacon, tomato, and

	avocado.
DAY 4	LETTUCE - WRAPPED BURGER INGREDIENTS FOR LETTUCE - WRAPPED BURGER i. 70g grounded pork ii. Two slices of bacon (50g) iii. One large lettuce leaf iv. One slice tomato v. 1 cup of fresh toddler spinach vi. 1 Tablespoon of mayonnaise COOKING INSTRUCTIONS 1. Fry by dipping the bacon in oil that is being heated in a very neat frying pan until its crispy. Form a hamburger patty with the ground pork. Then fry within the leftover bacon grease. Cook on both ends until its chefs properly. 2. Add the spinach to the remaining oil within the frying pan and cook till wilted. three. Add the tomato, spinach, mayonnaise, patty and bacon in a big lettuce leaf, fold and make a burger.

DAY 5	GRILLED COD AND SHRIMPS
	INGREDIENTS FOR GRILLED COD AND SHRIMPS
	i. Two cod fillet
	ii. 1 Tablespoon of lemon juice
	iii. Two tablespoons of olive oil
	iv. Two garlic cloves
	v. Eight cherry tomatoes
	vi. 200g shrimps
	vii. 2 stems fresh parsley
	viii. Two garlic cloves
	COOKING INSTRUCTIONS
	1. Finely chop the garlic and parsley.
	2. Melt the butter in a pan and encompass the garlic. Cook for few seconds and puts the cod and shrimp in the pan. Add the chopped parsley. Cook the shrimps for few mins until it turns orange. Cook the cod for two minutes on every side, be cautious not to interrupt it aside while turning it over. Include the tomatoes to the pan and fry with the shrimps for about one minute till it's far soft.
	three. Add the lemon juice. Then it's far set to be eaten.
DAY 6	ARUGULA CAESAR SALAD AND VEGETABLES

	INGREDIENTS FOR ARUGULA CAESAR SALAD AND VEGETABLES i. Three leaves of iceberg lettuce ii. Two asparagus iii. 40g arugula iv. Four broccoli florets v. 5-6 slices cucumber vi. half of avocado vii. 1 / 2 tomato One part of Caesar dressing COOKING INSTRUCTIONS 1. Place some water to boil and cook dinner the broccoli and asparagus until it is smooth 2. Shred the arugula and iceberg lettuce and vicinity into a bowl 3. Chop the avocado, cucumber, and tomato. Then positioned the entirety into a plate and cowl with the dressing
DAY 7	FLUFFY OMELET AND VEGETABLES INGREDIENTS i. half zucchini ii. 1 / 2 cup of fresh spinach iii. half of small cucumber iv. One hard-boiled egg

v. 1 serving basil Vinaigrette

COOKING INSTRUCTIONS

1. Using a cabbage shredder, slice the zucchini and cucumber thinly

2. Slice the spinach and reduce the egg into four

three. Place everything right into a plate and pour the dressing

DINNER

DAY 1	ARUGULA SALAD WITH BASIL VINAIGRETTE
	INGREDIENTS FOR ARUGULA SALAD WITH BASIL VINAIGRETTE
	i. 40g arugula
	ii. five to six slices of cucumber
	iii. 1 / 2 tomato
	iv. Two slices prosciutto
	v. Three broccoli florets
	vi. 1 serving basil Vinaigrette
	COOKING INSTRUCTIONS
	1. When water is boiling upload the broccoli to it. Cook, until it's far soft and cool, relaxed beneath bloodless water.
	2. Mix all the elements in a cooking container, and you're set.

| DAY 2 | BROCCOLI AND ROSEMARY CHICKEN |
| | INGREDIENTS FOR BROCCOLI AND ROSEMARY CHICKEN |

DAY 2

BROCCOLI AND ROSEMARY CHICKEN

INGREDIENTS FOR BROCCOLI AND ROSEMARY CHICKEN

i. One boneless bird leg

ii. one-quarter tablespoon of salt

iii. half of tablespoon of rosemary

iv. 1 Tablespoon of olive oil

v. 1/3 broccoli head

vi. one-quarter tablespoon of black pepper

vii. Two tablespoons of water

COOKING INSTRUCTIONS

1. Cut the chicken leg into bite-length pieces, then sprinkle salt and pepper on pinnacle of it. Separate the broccoli into florets.

2. In a cast-iron pan, permit the olive oil to get heated, and upload the hen to the rosemary. Fry for three minutes to crisp up the chook pores and skin and turn the bird around. Then continue to add the prepared broccoli florets, with that you can prepare dinner for two minutes blending the components, then inside the water, cowl it and allow the steam of the water to cook the broccoli for 2 minutes. Then scoop it and serve to your people.

DAY 3	ROASTED ROSEMARY PORK INGREDIENTS FOR ROASTED ROSEMARY PORK i. 500g boneless roast beef ii. 1 Tablespoon of olive oil iii. 1 Tablespoon of salt iv. 1 Tablespoon of black pepper v. 1 Tablespoon of rosemary COOKING INSTRUCTIONS 1 Preheat the oven in a temperature of 200C/400F. 2. Gently rubdown the salt, black pepper, salt, and rosemary into the beef roast, then placed it on a baking tray wrapped in bakery paper. 3. Put it within the oven and cook for one hour. Remove it, and permit it cool for 5 to ten mins. Slice and serve.
DAY 4	KALE BEEF AND VEGETABLES WRAPPED INGREDIENTS FOR KALE BEEF AND VEGETABLES WRAPPED i. half of avocado ii. 1 / 2 tomato iii. One portion of Caesar dressing iv. One massive kale leaf

	v. 1/8 purple onion vi. 100g thinly sliced beef vii. one-quarter tablespoon of pepper, salt, and garlic powder viii. 1 Tablespoon of olive oil COOKING INSTRUCTIONS 1. Trim the stem of the kale leaf cautiously to enable you to roll the leaf to make a sandwich. 2. Chop the avocado, tomato, and red onion. three. Place a saucepan with olive oil on a cooker and include the sliced red meat into the pan. Sprinkle the garlic powder, pepper, and salt and cook very well for 1 to 2 minutes. four. Scoop the Caesar dressing over the complete leaf. On one of the ceases, upload all of the toppings and roll the leaf into a wrap carefully. You can employ the aluminum foil to maintain it from rolling away.
DAY 5	EGG IN MINI SKILLET INGREDIENTS FOR EGG IN MINI SKILLET i. Two slices of bacon ii. 1 / 2 avocado iii. Two eggs

	iv. 1 / 2 tomato
	v. One okra
	vi. Three boiled broccoli
	vii. Sprinkle pepper, parsley, and salt
	COOKING INSTRUCTIONS
	1. Fry the bacon till it is crispy in a mini skillet of 6 inches. Chop the bacon into bits. Dice the avocado and tomato and slice the okra into some portions
	2. Using the same mini skillet, crack the eggs open into the bacon grease, cowl, and cook dinner on low heat till it cooks properly. Top it with the bacon bits, avocado, broccoli, okra, and tomato. Sprinkle salt, parsley, and pepper over it,
DAY 6	MUSHROOMS, BROCCOLI AND BACON MEAL INGREDIENTS FOR MUSHROOMS, BROCCOLI AND BACON MEAL i. 8og of broccoli ii. Four brown mushrooms iii. Three portions of bacon iv. one-quarter tablespoon of salt v. half tablespoon of rosemary vi. one-quarter tablespoon of garlic powder vii. A pinch of black pepper COOKING INSTRUCTIONS

	1. Boil little water in a pot and cook dinner the broccoli until it is soft. 2. Sprinkle salt over the bacon pieces and reduce into 1cm peeps. 3. Cut the mushrooms into six portions. 4. Fry the bacon in a pan for one minute and include the mushrooms. Add the rosemary to the broccoli, then blend the entirety, sprinkle the garlic powder, and black pepper on it.
DAY 7	RADISHES AND ROSEMARY SHRIMPS INGREDIENTS FOR RADISHES AND ROSEMARY SHRIMPS i. Five radishes ii. 1 Tablespoon olive oil iii. 1 Tablespoon of rosemary iv. Ten shrimps v. Three broccoli florets vi. half tablespoon salt and pepper COOKING INSTRUCTIONS 1. Boil some water in a pot and upload the broccoli then cook dinner until it tenders. 2. Put a frying pan with olive oil on a cooker to heat it, then include the radishes to an aspect and the shrimps to every other aspect, then sprinkle the salt, rosemary, and

	pepper and cook for few mins. The radishes should be crunchy and soft, and you must make certain the shrimps turn orange. Three. Put the whole thing in a plate and experience it.

DESSERT

DAY 1	LOW CARB BREAD INGREDIENTS FOR LOW CARB BREAD i. Four tablespoons of easily grounded almond meal ii. one-quarter tablespoon of baking soda iii. One huge egg iv. Two tablespoons of water v. Two tablespoons of olive oil vi. 1 / 4 tablespoon of salt COOKING INSTRUCTIONS 1. In a shallow small microwave-secure container, whisk the flour, salt, and baking soda together. 2. Make a hollow inside the center and destroy an egg open into it, then whisk well. Add inside the olive oil and water at the same time as blending. three. When it forms very well, start making large circles together with your fork to comprise the flour blend.

four. Mix thoroughly, including the edges and sides, then use a spatula to make certain it mixes flawlessly.

five. Tap the bowl down on the counter to ensure the combination settle.

6. Microwave for ninety seconds on high heat or heat until the center is properly cooked.

7. If you're baking it, employ a greased glass dish and bake at 325F convection for 20 mins, then use a spatula across the facets to separate it from the container.

eight. Pop right into a toaster for three-4 mins until it's miles crispy and geared up to eat.

DAY 2	THE MEDITERRANEAN ALMOND BUTTER BURGER
	INGREDIENTS FOR THE MEDITERRANEAN ALMOND BUTTER BURGER
	i. Two tablespoons of grounded turkey
	ii. 1 Tablespoon of apple cider
	iii. Vinegar
	iv. One large egg
	v. half cup of almond butter crunchy and unsweetened
	vi. 1 Tablespoon of black pepper
	vii. 1 Tablespoon of fish sauce
	viii. 1 Tablespoon of turmeric
	ix. 1 / 2 tablespoon of garlic salt

COOKING INSTRUCTIONS

1. Start by way of preheating the oven till it gets to 400F.

2. Mix all the listed ingredients above right into a massive bowl until well-formed, then gently grease a large baking sheet.

three. Shape into ten patties like four oz every then area at the baking sheet.

four. Bake for 20-25 mins.

| DAY 3 | MEDITERRANEAN MEAL WITH GREEN SAUCE |

MEDITERRANEAN MEAL WITH GREEN SAUCE

INGREDIENTS FOR MEDITERRANEAN MEAL WITH GREEN SAUCE

i. 1 cup of child spinach

ii. 1 cup of arugula

iii. 1 cup of parsley

iv. Five medium of garlic cloves

v. Five tablespoons of hemp hearts

vi. 1 cup of olive oil

vii. Five slices bacon

viii. Two eggs

ix. 20 asparagus guidelines

x. Salt

xi. Pepper

| | COOKING INSTRUCTIONS |
| | |

COOKING INSTRUCTIONS

1. To make a green sauce integrate child spinach, parsley, garlic cloves, arugula, and olive oil right into a blender and mix the components on low speed until it's far properly-fashioned and easy and set aside.

2. On a sheet pan, arrange your bacon chops into rings and prepare it into circles.

three. Pop the sheet pan into the oven then set to a temperature of 320F. When the oven is at excessive temperature, take away the sheet pan from the oven and suit the four asparagus suggestions into every bacon ring.

4. Move your bacon rings together if essential after which spoil two eggs in among them.

five. Add your already made green sauce, sprinkle little pepper and salt and go back to the oven for 20minutes.

6. Remove from the oven and enjoy!

DAY 4

ASPARAGUS, SAUCE AND AVOCADO BOAT MEAL

INGREDIENTS FOR ASPARAGUS, SAUCE AND AVOCADO BOAT MEAL

i. Asparagus, sausage and avocado boat

ii. 60g sausage

	iii. 1 or 2 asparagus iv. 1 Tablespoon olive oil v. half of avocado vi. 70g Tuna vii. 1/4 cup of wilted spinach viii. 1 Tablespoon of mayonnaise ix. Pinch salt and pepper COOKING INSTRUCTIONS 1. Place a small frying pan on fireplace to warmth the olive oil and fry the sausages and asparagus until its chefs well then transfer to a plate. 2. Spoon out the inner of the avocado and put it in a bowl with the Tuna, mayonnaise, wilted spinach and salt and pepper. Put the avocado shell with it and area it on a plate.
DAY 5	VEGETABLES BROCHETTES AND CHICKEN INGREDIENTS FOR VEGETABLES BROCHETTES AND CHICKEN i. One boneless bird leg (300g) ii. four Asparagus iii. 1 Tablespoon of rosemary iv. Ten cherry tomatoes

	v. Five garlic cloves vi. half of tablespoon of onion powder vii. 1 Tablespoon of salt and pepper viii. 1 Tablespoon of olive oil ix. 1 Tablespoon lemon juice from a lemon x. One huge Asian COOKING INSTRUCTIONS 1. Preheat the oven to 210C / 420F. 2. Chop the chook leg into biteable portions. Slice the lengthy green onion into 12 to 14 pieces. Then cut the asparagus into 4. 3. Combine all the substances into a cooking bowl and blend. Skewer the vegetables and fowl on the brochettes. 4. Place within the oven and bake for 20 mins.
DAY 6	SESAME SALAD AND CHICKEN BROCHETTES INGREDIENTS FOR SESAME SALAD AND CHICKEN BROCHETTES i. Three chook and vegetable brochettes ii. Three lettuce leaves iii. One tomato slice iv. One portion of sesame dressing v. 1/4 avocado COOKING INSTRUCTIONS

	1. Cut the lettuce into portions size biteable. Scoop out the avocado flesh and cube it, chop the tomato into few portions. Add the sesame dressing and coat thoroughly. 2. Add the brochettes to a plate with the salad and experience!
DAY 7	PORK OMELET AND SPINACH INGREDIENTS FOR PORK OMELET AND SPINACH i. One sausage ii. 1 cup of sparkling spinach iii. 1/4 crimson pepper iv. Two garlic cloves v. Two tablespoons of olive oil vi. 1/ 4 tablespoon of pepper, garlic powder, and salt vii. 1/4 tablespoon of parsley viii. Six eggs COOKING INSTRUCTIONS 1. Crush the sausage. Chop the purple pepper and finely chop the garlic. 2. In a massive nonstick frying pan, prepare dinner the sausage and add the olive oil. Add the crimson pepper, spinach, and garlic to the pan and cook dinner for 1 or 2 minutes until it is soft. three. Break the eggs open in a massive bowl, add the

spices and combine with a whisk for two minutes.

four. Pour the battered egg to the pan, then cowl and permit it to prepare dinner on a low warmth for 4 to five minutes.

5. When the pinnacle of the omelet is ready, slide the omelet to a plate and reduce into two you may eat 1/2 nowadays and the opposite the next day.

SNACK

DAY 1	CHICKEN GRILLED THIGH WITH ZUCCHINI SALAD
	INGREDIENTS FOR CHICKEN GRILLED THIGH WITH ZUCCHINI SALAD
	i. 1/4 Zucchini
	ii. 1/4 purple pepper
	iii. Five basil leaves
	iv. One garlic clove
	v. One fowl thigh with a skin of (75g)
	vi. 50g Swiss chard

	vii. 1/2 tablespoon of salt and pepper
	viii. 1 Tablespoon of olive oil
	ix. 1 Tablespoon of vinegar
	x. one-quarter tomato
	COOKING INSTRUCTIONS
	1. Using a peeler, peel the zucchini in a lengthwise shape to make lengthy ribbons. Cut the red pepper in 1/2. Dice the tomato. Slice the Swiss chard. Finely chop the basil leaves and garlic cloves.
	2. Mix all of the above substances with olive oil, salt, pepper, and vinegar together in a bowl and location it on a plate.
	3. Spray the salt and pepper over the hen thigh. Preheat the oil in a cast-iron pan and location the hen breast skin aspect down and prepare dinner till it is miles crispy. Flip it around, cook a few more mins until nicely cooked, then area on the plate with the salad.
DAY 2	GRILLED SALMON AND GREEN BEANS AND RADISHES
	INGREDIENTS FOR GRILLED SALMON AND GREEN BEANS AND RADISHES
	i. 150g of salmon fillet
	ii. 3 Tablespoon of olive oil

iii. one-quarter tablespoon of salt, black pepper, and dill

iv. 1 Tablespoon of lemon juice

v. 1 Tablespoon of rosemary

vi. Five radishes

vii. Pinch of salt, garlic powder, and pepper

viii. One garlic clove

ix. 50g green beans

COOKING INSTRUCTIONS

1. Rub the salmon with oil, salt, pepper and dill.

2. Place a nonstick frying pan carefully and cook on both aspects for two to 3 minutes until it's miles perfectly cooked via. Once nicely cooked, add the lemon juice on top of the salmon

3. Finely chop the garlic clove. Place the green beans to a boil and prepare dinner for 5 to six mins. Take out of the water into a pan accompany the olive oil and the finely chopped garlic. Sprinkle the salt and pepper over it and prepare dinner in the frying pan until the garlic receives crunchy.

four. Put a frying pan with olive oil on a cooker to heat the olive oil, then include the rosemary and radishes. Then mix cook for 4-five mins till it is miles crispy. Sprinkle the salt and pepper on it once more.

DAY 3	COCONUT FLOUR PORRIDGE

COCONUT FLOUR PORRIDGE

INGREDIENTS FOR COCONUT FLOUR PORRIDGE

i. 2 tablespoons coconut flour

ii. 2 tablespoons golden flax meal

iii. 3/four cup water

iv. Pinch of salt

v. 1 large egg beaten

vi. 2 teaspoons butter or ghee

vii. 1 tablespoon heavy cream or coconut milk

viii. 1 tablespoon Low carb brown sugar or your favorite sweetener

Instructions

1. Start by measuring the first four substances right into a saucepan or a small pot. Allow it to warmness for approximately 5mins and stir. When it starts to simmer, flip it down to medium-low and whisk till it starts off evolved to thicken.

2. Remove the coconut flour porridge from heat and add the crushed egg, half at a time, even as whisking the mixture continuously. Place it back on the heat and keep whisking until the porridge thickens.

three. Remove the pan from the warmth and maintain to whisk for about 30 seconds before including the butter, cream and sweetener.

4. Garnish it along with your favored toppings.

MEDITERRANEAN BAKED OMELET

INGREDIENTS FOR MEDITERRANEAN BAKED OMELET

i. half lb. Browned and crumbled sausage

ii. 8 massive eggs

iii. 1/2 cup heavy whipping cream

iv. 1 cup shredded Cheddar cheese

v. Salt, pepper, and other seasonings, to flavor good

Instructions

1. Preheat oven to 380°F. Spray a 7x11-inch baking dish with non-stick cooking spray.

2. Place the cooked and crumbled sausage flippantly within the prepared pan.

3. In a big bowl, whisk the eggs, heavy cream, cheese, and any preferred seasonings until they're nicely combined. Pour the egg combination frivolously over the sausage.

four. Bake for half-hour or until the edges start to brown. Then your Mediterranean omelet is prepared to be served.

| DAY 4 | CHEESY BACON OMELET |

	INGREDIENTS FOR CHEESY BACON OMELET i. 3 Large Eggs ii. 30 g Cheddar Cheese Grated iii. 2 Slices bacon Instructions 1. Heat a frying pan to medium-high heat, wait until you can experience the heat by soaring your hand five centimeters above the pan. 2. Place the bacon in the pan and prepare dinner till crispy. three. In an everyday bowl, whisk the eggs. 4. Remove the bacon along with as a good deal grease as possible. Pour it in the whisked eggs. five. Cook for approximately 3-four minutes, area the cheese and bacon on one half of the Omelet and turn one side over onto the cheese and bacon. Cook for every other 1-2 minutes.
DAY 5	MEDITERRANEAN FATHEAD PIZZA INGREDIENTS FOR MEDITERRANEAN FATHEAD PIZZA i. 1 half of cup Mozzarella cheese (shredded) ii. 2 tbsp Cream cheese (reduce into cubes) iii. 2 large Egg (beaten)

iv. 1/3 cup Coconut flour

v. One out of pepperoni, peppers, cherry tomatoes, olives, floor/mince red meat, mushrooms, herbs.

Instructions

1. Preheat your oven to 425 levels F (218 tiers C). Start to line a baking sheet, pizza pan with the necessary parchment paper.

2. Mix the diced mozzarella and cubed cream cheese in a massive bowl. Microwave for ninety seconds, stirring halfway through. Stir once more at the stop till nicely incorporated.

three. Stir inside the crushed eggs and coconut flour. You must ensure that you knead the flour with your hands until a dough form. If the dough turns into hard before fully combined, you could microwave for 10-15 seconds to melt it.

4. Spread the dough onto the covered baking pan to 1/4" or 1/3" thickness, the use of your arms or a rolling pin over a piece of parchment. However, the rolling pin works better when you have one. You must ensure to use a toothpick or the tinge of your spoon or fork to poke lots of holes all through the crust to prevent bubbling and to make sure it cooks flippantly.

five. Bake for six minutes. Poke more holes in any locations wherein you notice bubbles forming. Bake for three-7 extra mins, till golden brown.

6. Once cooked, cast off from the oven and add all the toppings you want. Make positive any meat that you'll be adding inside the topping is already cooked as this time it goes back into the oven simply to warmness up the toppings and melt the cheese. Bake again at 220C/425F for simply 5 minutes.

DAY 6	**LOADED CAULIFLOWER CASSEROLE**

LOADED CAULIFLOWER CASSEROLE

INGREDIENTS FOR LOADED CAULIFLOWER CASSEROLE

i. 1-pound cauliflower

ii. 4 oz bitter cream

iii. 1 cup cheddar cheese (grated or shredded)

iv. 2 slices bacon cooked and crumbled

v. 2 tablespoons chives snipped

vi. 3 tablespoons butter

vii. one-quarter teaspoon garlic powder

viii. Salt and black pepper

Instructions

1. To begin with, cut the cauliflower into florets, then placed them right into a microwave-safe bowl. Add two tablespoons of water and cover with dangle film.

2. Add the cauliflower to a meals processor and system till it turns into fluffy. Add the butter, garlic powder, and

	buttercream, then technique until it resembles the consistency of mashed potatoes. three. Top the loaded cauliflower with the final cheese, closing chives and bacon. Put lower back into the microwave to melt the cheese or place the cauliflower under the broiler for a couple of minutes.
DAY 7	BROCCOLI FRITTERS WITH CHEDDAR CHEESE INGREDIENTS FOR BROCCOLI FRITTERS WITH CHEDDAR CHEESE i. 1 small broccoli head or 1/2 large one ii. 1 egg (beaten) iii. A handful of grated cheddar cheese iv. 2 Tbsp oat fiber or almond flour, or powdered beef rinds v. 1Tbsps avocado oil or any of your favored oil Instructions 1. First, loosely chop your broccoli and then steam gently for a few minutes till it's far tender. Drain any excess water and dry with paper towels if wet. 2. On a cutting board, reduce the cooked broccoli into very small pieces. 3. Then area it in a bowl and add the egg. Using a spoon, mix the egg via the broccoli mix as plenty as you could. 4. Heat a few avocado oil in a pan. The oil has to be

enough to cowl the bottom, but no extra.

5. Cook on one facet till the cheese at the top of the patty starts off evolved to soften and the bottom is crusty brown.

five. Remove from the oil and permit take a seat on a few paper towels for a couple of minutes to soak up the grease, earlier than dishing up. You can serve it topped with an egg or with a dipping sauce.

2. Second Week

BREAKFAST

<table>
<tr><td>

DAY 1

</td><td>

ROASTED CAULIFLOWER WITH BACON AND GREEN ONIONS

INGREDIENTS FOR ROASTED CAULIFLOWER WITH BACON AND GREEN ONIONS

i. 1 head cauliflower

ii. three slices of bacon

iii. 4 green onion sliced into half of inch portions

iv. 1 tablespoon olive oil

v. one-quarter teaspoon salt

vi. one-quarter teaspoon freshly ground black pepper

Instructions

1. Preheat your oven to 400 levels F.

2. Cut the cauliflower into chew sized pieces. Slice the red onions the use of simplest the white and mild parts. Slice the bacon into chunks.

3. Toss the cauliflower, green onion, and bacon with the olive oil and unfold on a sheet pan. Season with the salt and pepper.

four. Cook the cauliflower 10 mins, stir, then cook for 15 mins greater or until the cauliflower begins to brown.

five. Place under the broiler for a few minutes if you

</td></tr>
</table>

	want greater caramelizing. Add extra salt and pepper to flavor. Serve.
DAY 2	COCONUT CHICKEN CURRY INGREDIENTS FOR COCONUT CHICKEN CURRY i. 2 tbsp Olive oil ii. half huge onion (chopped) iii. 1 lb. chook thighs (cut into bit) iv. 14 diced tomatoes or five ounce of diced tomatoes (this must be well drained for best result) v. 7 ounces of coconut cream (the entire cream component skimmed from a 14-ozcan) vi. 1/4 cup bird broth vii. four cloves garlic (minced) viii. 1 half of tbsp curry powder ix. 1 tsp floor ginger x. 1 tsp paprika xi. 1/2 tsp sea salt Instructions 1. Heat the oil that you want to use in a very large saucepan over medium warmth. Add the onion and allow

to cook dinner for approximately 7 to 10 mins, until it's miles nicely browned.

2. Push the onion to the facet and growth warmth to medium excessive. Add some other tablespoon of oil and the fowl in a single layer.

three. Add the diced tomatoes, coconut cream, chicken broth, garlic, curry powder, floor ginger, paprika, and sea salt. Stir everything together and alter the salt to taste.

4. You must ensure that you let the mixture which you have put on fire to boil, then reduce the warmth. Cover the saucepan which you are the use of and provide the sauce proper time to simmer, permit's say for approximately 15 to twenty minutes till the chicken is cooked thru and the sauce is thick.

five. Your coconut chook curry is prepared to be served with cauliflower rice or any of your appropriate dish.

DAY 3

MEDITERRANEAN SALMON FILLED AVOCADO

INGREDIENTS FOR MEDITERRANEAN SALMON FILLED AVOCADO

i. Small-medium or 1 huge avocado, with its seed removed (2 hundred g / 7.1 oz)

ii. 2 small or one massive salmon fillet (220 g / 7. eight oz)

iii. 1 large purple onion, that is correctly chopped and

diced (ninety g / 3. five oz) cup soured cream or crème fraiche or mayonnaise,

iv. 2 tbsp fresh lemon juice

v. Salt

vi. Freshly ground black pepper

vii. 1 tbsp coconut oil

viii. 1-2 tbsp freshly chopped dill

ix. Lemon wedges for garnish

Instructions

1 Preheat the oven to two hundred F / 400 F. Place the salmon fillets on a baking tray coated with parchment paper.

2. Drizzle with melted ghee or coconut oil, season with salt and pepper and 1 tablespoon of sparkling lemon juice. Place this inside your oven and ensure that you bake this recipe for 20-25 minutes at least.

2 When finished, get rid of it from the oven and let it settle down for five-10 minutes.

4 Squeeze in more lemon juice and season with salt and pepper to flavor. Scoop the middle of the avocado out leaving about an inch of the avocado flesh. Cut the scooped avocado into small portions.

5 Place the chopped avocado into the bowl with salmon and mix till properly combined.

6 Fill each avocado 1/2 with the salmon & avocado

	combination, upload lemon and experience!
DAY 4	MEDITERRANEAN CARBONARA INGREDIENTS FOR MEDITERRANEAN CARBONARA i. 2 lbs. boneless skinless fowl thighs (reduce into chew-sized portions) ii. ½ tsp garlic powder iii. Salt and pepper to taste iv. 6 slices cooked bacon (crumbled) v. 1 tbsp bacon grease vi. ½ cup onion chopped vii. 2 tsp minced garlic viii. 1 cup heavy whipping cream ix. 1 cup hen broth x. 1 crushed egg (optional) xi. ⅓ cup Parmesan cheese (grated) xii. 1 tsp Italian seasoning xiii. 1 tbsp fresh chopped basil xiv. 2-3 cups clean spinach Instructions 1. Cook the bacon until crispy and then fall apart into pieces. 2. Place 1 tbsp of the bacon grease in a huge skillet over

medium-excessive heat.

3. Add the chicken to the skillet and sprinkle with the garlic powder in addition to salt and pepper to flavor.

four. In the equal skillet, upload the ½ cup of chopped onion and prepare dinner for a couple of minutes until they come to be tender.

five. Add the minced garlic, and sauté for some other 30 seconds.

6. Whisk the heavy whipping the cream and the fowl broth, cautiously scraping the bits off the lowest of the skillet.

7. This is optional; put the crushed egg in a very small bowl. Carefully movement the sauce into the egg while you're nonetheless whisking it.

8. Ensure to mix in the parmesan cheese, chopped basil, and Italian seasoning.

9. Toss within the crumbled bacon, and 2-3 cups of fresh spinach. Cook until the spinach has begun to wilt.

10. Add the chicken back into the skillet and toss to coat inside the sauce. Sprinkle in extra salt and pepper to flavor.

eleven. Simmer the aggregate for three-five mins longer and serve.

DAY 5	MEDITERRANEAN CHICKEN QUESADILLA

INGREDIENTS FOR MEDITERRANEAN CHICKEN QUESADILLA

i. Serves: 1 quesadilla

ii. Ingredients

iii. 1½ Cups Mozzarella Cheese

iv. 1½ Cups Cheddar Cheese

v. 1 Cup Cooked Chicken

vi. ¼ Cup Bell Pepper

vii. ¼ Cup Diced Tomato

viii. ⅛ Cup Green Onion

Instructions

1. Preheat your oven to 400 F (200 °C). Then, cover a pizza pan with Parchment Paper. Mix the cheese collectively in a bowl, then evenly spread them over the parchment paper in a circle form.

2. Bake the cheese shell for at least, five mins. Remove any more oil from the cheese.

3. Place the fowl over half of the cheese shell. Then upload the sliced peppers, diced tomato and the chopped green onion.

4. Fold the cheese shell in half of over the chook and veggies. Press it firmly, then positioned it inside the oven for every other four- five minutes.

five. Serve with sour cream, salsa and guacamole. Garnish with Chopped Fresh Basil, Parsley or Cilantro.

<table>
<tr><td>DAY 6</td><td>

MEDITERRANEAN RIBEYE STEAK WITH OVEN-ROASTED VEGETABLE

INGREDIENTS FOR MEDITERRANEAN RIBEYE STEAK WITH OVEN-ROASTED VEGETABLE

i. 1 lbs. broccoli

ii. 1 Whole garlic

iii. 10 oz. Cherry tomatoes

iv. three tbsp olive oil

v. 1 tbsp dried thyme or dried oregano or dried basil

vi. 1½ lbs. ribeye steaks

vii. Salt and pepper

viii. Anchovy butter

ix. 1 oz. Anchovies

x. 5 oz. Butter, at room temperature

xi. 1 tbsp lemon juice

xii. Salt and pepper

Instructions

1. Chop the anchovy fillets and mix them with butter, lemon juice, salt and pepper. Then set it aside.

2. Make certain your meat is out of the fridge if you want to get it to room temperature earlier than cooking it.

3. Preheat your oven to 450°F (225°C). Grease a huge roasting pan and location all the vegetables in a single

</td></tr>
</table>

	layer. Season and drizzle olive oil on top.
	4. Brush the beef with olive oil and season with salt and pepper. Fry speedy on high heat in a frying pan.
	5. Then, take away the pan from the oven and make room for the beef amongst the veggies.
	6. Lower the warmth to 400°F (200°C) and location the pan lower back inside the oven for a couple of minutes up to 10 or 15, depending on how you like your meat - rare, medium or nicely-accomplished.
	7. Remove from the oven and region a dollop of anchovy butter on each piece of meat. Serve immediately and experience your meals!
DAY 7	MEDITERRANEAN CHICKEN FRIED STEAK AND MUSHROOM GRAVY
	INGREDIENTS FOR MEDITERRANEAN CHICKEN FRIED STEAK AND MUSHROOM GRAVY
	i. three oz of pork rinds, overwhelmed inside the meal's processor
	ii. half teaspoon onion powder
	iii. half of teaspoon garlic powder
	iv. 1 teaspoon salt
	v. 1 teaspoon freshly floor black pepper
	vi. 2 Eggs(beaten)
	vii. 4-ounce small steaks or cube steaks

viii. 2 tablespoons of butter

ix. 8 oz. Baby Bella Mushrooms, sliced

x. 1/2 cup heavy cream

xi. 1 1/2 cup beef broth

xii. half of teaspoon xanthan gum

xiii. Salt and pepper to flavor

xiv. Oil if pan-frying

xv. Oil spray if air frying

xvi. Air fryer

Instructions

1. To prepare the dredge station: Combine all the crushed pork rinds, onion powder, garlic powder, salt and pepper in a shallow bowl. Stir properly and mix them.

2. Add the beaten eggs in every other shallow bowl.

3. To dredge the dice steaks. First, coat them within the egg then start to coat them with the pork rind combination.

four. Do this for every dice steak and set it aside.

5. If air frying, spray the internal of the air fryer basket with cooking spray.

6. Place dice steaks within the air fryer and prepare dinner at 400 F for 15 minutes. After that begin to show the steaks halfway thru the cooking time. Remove from the air fryer and set aside.

7. To maintain them warm, region them on a sheet tray

and placed them in oven, at lowest temperature (normally 200F) even as the alternative dice steak prepare dinner.

7. Continue with the alternative two steaks.

8. While the steaks are nevertheless cooking, make certain to make the mushroom gravy.

9. In a big skillet over medium heat, cook dinner the mushrooms within the butter until the mushrooms are tender. This will take about five to eight minutes.

10. Add inside the heavy cream and beef broth.

eleven. Whisk within the xanthan gum and convey to boil for a few minutes to allow thicken.

12. Season with salt and pepper to flavor.

13. Serve the minute steaks crowned with the mushroom gravy.

LUNCH

DAY 1	LOW CARBS CUBE STEAK AND EGGS

INGREDIENTS FOR LOW CARBS CUBE STEAK AND EGGS

i. 8 ounces cube steak

ii. 4 huge eggs

iii. 2 tablespoon butter (divided)

iv. 2-ounce cheddar cheese

v. 8 ounces asparagus trimmed

vi. Salt and black pepper

Instructions

1. Preparation: Trim the asparagus and vicinity it in a microwaveable dish. Add 1 tablespoon water and cover with plastic wrap.

2. Cube Steak: Season both facets of the cube steaks with salt and black pepper. Heat a medium cast-iron skillet over medium heat. When hot, upload 1 tablespoon of butter and swirl to coat the bottom. Add the pro cube steaks and prepare dinner 3 - four half minutes consistent with side (or longer) depending on your selected stage of doneness. Remove the cooked cube steaks to an area and tent lightly with foil.

3. Cheesy Scrambled Eggs: While the steaks are cooking, region a medium non-stick pan over medium warmth. Crack four eggs right into a medium bowl and add 2 ounces of grated cheese. Mix with a fork. When the pan

	is warm, add 1 tablespoon of butter and swirl to coat the pan. Add the egg mixture to the pan and depart it on my own for a few moments whilst its chefs on the lowest. Gently scrape the boiled egg to the center of the pan with a rubber spatula. Break up the center with the spatula and flip off the warmth. five. Serve: Place one dice steak on each plate, add half of the asparagus and season it with salt and pepper. Place half of the cheesy eggs on top and season with salt and pepper.
DAY 2	PALEO SHRIMP ALFREDO WITH ARTICHOKES HEARTS INGREDIENTS FOR PALEO SHRIMP ALFREDO WITH ARTICHOKES HEARTS i. 4 medium zucchini ii. 2 tsp sea salt divided iii. 2 tbsp ghee or coconut oil for AIP, divided iv. 1 onion chopped v. three garlic cloves minced vi. 1 14-ouncescan coconut cream vii. 1 tbsp lemon juice viii. 1 tbsp dietary yeast ix. 1 tsp garlic powder x. 1/2 tsp floor black pepper omit for AIP

xi. one-quarter cup chopped parsley

xii. 1 lb. raw shrimp peeled and deveined

xiii. 1 14oz can of Reese Quartered Artichoke Hearts (drained and moisture squeezed out)

Instructions

1. Use a vegetable peeler or spiralizer to slice the zucchini into noodles.

2. Place the zucchini noodles in a colander over a bowl and toss with 1 tsp of sea salt.

three. Let this sit down for half-hour to sweat the zucchini. Start cooking the shrimp and the sauce at the same time as the zucchini sits.

four. Pat dry the shrimp with a paper towel and warmth 1 tbsp of ghee in a massive skillet over medium-excessive warmth.

five. Add shrimp in a single layer and pan-fry for two minutes on each facet.

6. Remove the shrimp from the pan and set aside.

7. Heat some other tbsp of ghee within the equal skillet.

8. Add onion and garlic and sauté for three-4 mins till the onions are translucent.

9. Add coconut cream, lemon juice, dietary yeast, 1 tsp sea salt, garlic powder, and ground black pepper.

10. Once the sauce starts off evolved to boil, reduce the warmth to medium low to simmer for 20 minutes till

reduced.

11. Drain the zucchini and wrap in a paper towel to squeeze out the moisture.

12. Stir in Reese Quartered Artichoke Hearts, zucchini noodles, and parsley, and permit everything simmer for five greater mins at the same time as stirring frequently.

13. Turn off heat and stir in shrimp. Serve warm.

DAY 3	MEDITERRANEAN FRITTATA WITH FRESH SPINACH INGREDIENTS FOR MEDITERRANEAN FRITTATA WITH FRESH SPINACH i. 8 eggs ii. 1 cup heavy whipping cream iii. 1/3 Ib diced bacon iv. 1/three Ib sparkling spinach v. 2 tablespoon butter for frying vi. Salt and pepper Instructions 1.Preheat the oven to 350°F (175°C). Fry the bacon in butter till crispy. Then, add the spinach. 2. Whisk the eggs and cream collectively and pour into a greased baking dish. 3. Add the bacon, spinach and cheese on pinnacle and region within the middle of the oven.

four. Bake for 25–half-hour.

You can serve with shredded green or purple cabbage with a homemade dressing. Delicious!

MEDITERRANEAN ASIAN BEEF SALAD

INGREDIENTS FOR MEDITERRANEAN ASIAN BEEF SALAD

i. Sesame mayonnaise

ii. ¾ cup mayonnaise

iii. 1 tsp sesame oil

iv. ½ tbsp lime juice

v. Salt and pepper

vi. Beef

vii. 1 tbsp olive oil

viii. 1 tbsp fish sauce

ix. 1 tbsp grated sparkling ginger

x. 1 tsp chili flakes

xi. / lb ribeye steaks

xii. Salad

xiii. 3 oz. Cherry tomatoes

xiv. 2 oz. Cucumber

xv. three oz. Lettuce

xvi. ½ pink onion

xvii. sparkling cilantro

	xviii. 1 tsp sesame seeds xix. 2 scallions Instructions 1. To put together the sesame mayonnaise: blend the mayonnaise with the sesame oil and lime juice. Then season it with salt and pepper and set aside. 2. To prepare the pork: Mix all ingredients for the beef marinade and pour right into a plastic bag. Add the beef and marinate for 15 minutes or extra at room temperature. three. Chop all greens for the salad, besides the scallions, into bite-sized pieces. Divide it among plates. four. Heat a medium frying pan over medium heat. Add sesame seeds to the dry pan, and toast them for a couple of minutes, or until they're gently browned and fragrant. 5. Pat the meat dry on both aspects with paper towels. 6. Fry the scallions for a minute inside the identical pan. 7. Slice the beef, across the grain, into thin slices. Place red meat and scallions on pinnacle of the veggies. 8. Top with roasted sesame seeds and serve with a dollop of sesame mayonnaise on the aspect.
DAY 4	TUNA EGG SALAD INGREDIENTS FOR TUNA EGG SALAD

	i. 1/2 cup Mayonnaise ii. 1 tbsp Dijon mustard iii. 1 tbsp fresh parsley iv. half of tsp Paprika v. 3 5-oz. Can tuna (tired) vi. 1/4 cup Celery (finely chopped) vii. 2 tbsp Pickles (finely chopped) viii. 2 tbsp white onion (minced) ix. four huge difficult-boiled eggs (diced) x. Sea salt xi. Black pepper Instructions 1. In a medium bowl, use a fork to whisk together the mayo, mustard, parsley, and paprika, until easy. 2. Add the tuna, celery, pickles, and onions. Stir together, breaking aside any large pieces of tuna. 3. Fold in the diced eggs.
DAY 5	MEDITERRANEAN MUSHROOM OMELET INGREDIENTS FOR MEDITERRANEAN MUSHROOM OMELET For the egg mixture: i. 2 eggs ii. three tablespoon chopped mushrooms iii. 2 tablespoon sliced olives

	iv. 2 tablespoon cream cheese v. 1 tablespoon chopped sparkling coriander vi. 1 green chili, chopped vii. ⅛ teaspoon salt viii. ⅛ teaspoon pepper ix. 2 tablespoon ghee or butter x. ¼ cup cheddar cheese xi. Lettuce to serve Instructions 1. Whisk all ingredients of egg combination collectively. 2. Heat the ghee or butter in a pan. Pour the combination into a non-stick pan and fry for 2 mins on medium warmth. three. Then slide the omelet right into a large plate. Flip the omelet again to the pan and prepare dinner for every other two mins. 4. Sprinkle cheddar cheese and allow it to soften. Fold the omelet and serve with lettuce and olives.
DAY 6	MEDITERRANEAN CHEESE ROLL-UPS INGREDIENTS FOR MEDITERRANEAN CHEESE ROLL-UPS i. 8 oz. Cheddar cheese or provolone cheese or Edam cheese, in slices

	ii. 2 oz. Butter Instructions 1. Place the cheese slices on a huge reducing board. 1 2. Slice butter with a cheese slicer or reduce actually skinny portions with a knife. 3. Cover every cheese slice with butter and roll-up. Serve as a snack.
DAY 7	MEDITERRANEAN CHICKEN SOUP INGREDIENTS FOR MEDITERRANEAN CHICKEN SOUP i. 16 oz. cooked chook, diced (I used rotisserie) ii. 6 cups bone broth or unsalted chook broth iii. For the vegetable base iv. four tbsp butter, avocado oil, or olive oil v. 8 oz celery root, cubed (half of a large celeriac) vi. 1 cup celery, sliced (2-3 stalks) vii. 1/2 cup onion, diced (2 oz or half of a small onion) viii. 1/three cup carrot, roll cut (3 oz or 1 medium carrot) ix. 1 large garlic clove, sliced x. 1 tsp lemon zest xi. 1 whole bay leaf xii. 1 tbsp garlic herb seasoning mixture xiii. 2 tsp chook base (paste, granulated, or bouillon)

xiv. one-quarter cup dry white wine (or 2 tsp lemon juice combined with water)

xv. Salt and pepper.

Instructions

1. Dice the fowl. Then peel and reduce the vegetables.

2. Place a four-quart lidded pot over medium-excessive warmness. When it becomes hot, you should add the butter or oil (anyone you choose to use) and all the greens, lemon zest, and bay leaf. Stir to coat the substances.

3. Reduce warmth to medium and add the garlic herb seasoning mixture, the chicken base and wine (or lemon-water mixture).

4. Add the chicken broth and convey it to simply below a boil. Ensure you reduce the heat for the food to simmer and cook dinner till the greens are cooked through it all.

five. Add the chicken and salt and pepper to flavor and to make the soup greater savory.

DINNER

DAY 1	CHEESY CHICKEN
	INGREDIENTS FOR CHEESY CHICKEN
	i. 4 slices of pork loin joint,

	ii. 4 bird drumsticks, iii. Celtic sea salt, iv. Freshly ground bell pepper, v. half of shredded mozzarella cheese, chopped red meat mince for garnishing Instructions 1. Cook the pork loin joint till crispy for about eight mins in a skillet. Transfer the pork to a plate. 2. After, season the hen with the salt and pepper and prepare dinner inside the skillet for another 6 minutes, till each facet flip golden. 3. Sprinkle bird with the mozzarella cheese and prepare dinner until the cheese melts into the hen four. Then, crush the pork and unfold it at the hen and pinnacle with the beef mince. There you go, your cheesy meal is prepared!
DAY 2	MEDITERRANEAN QUESADILLA INGREDIENTS FOR MEDITERRANEAN QUESADILLA i. 1 sliced bell pepper, ii. 1 tbsp of more-virgin olive oil, iii. half faucet of Himalayan salt, iv. Shredded chicken thighs (2), v. 1 thinly-sliced avocado,

	vi. 1 shredded goat's cheese,
	vii. 1 Chester cheese
	Instructions
	1. First, preheat your oven to about 350° to 400° Celsius. Then in a skillet, heat the virgin olive oil. Add your pepper and salt and seasoning to the oil. Let it simmer until the pepper is soft. After, switch to a plate.
	2. In a bowl, stir both portions of cheese collectively. Then pour into the center of two baking sheets, even out the layers and shape right into a circle.
	3. Bake the cheese aggregate in the preheated oven till its edge becomes golden. Add the pepper aggregate, shredded hen and avocado slices to the combination in every baking sheet. After, use a spatula to fold the other aspect of the cheese over the aspect which has the fillings.
	4. Heat in the oven for another three to four mins and your dish is ready. Serve with garnishing of your choice.
DAY 3	MEDITERRANEAN QUESADILLA
	INGREDIENTS FOR MEDITERRANEAN QUESADILLA
	i. 1 sliced bell pepper,
	ii. 1 tbsp of more-virgin olive oil,
	iii. half faucet of Himalayan salt,

	iv. Shredded chicken thighs (2),
	v. 1 thinly-sliced avocado,
	vi. 1 shredded goat's cheese,
	vii. 1 Chester cheese
	Instructions
	1. First, preheat your oven to about 350° to 400° Celsius. Then in a skillet, heat the virgin olive oil. Add your pepper and salt and seasoning to the oil. Let it simmer until the pepper is soft. After, switch to a plate.
	2. In a bowl, stir both portions of cheese collectively. Then pour into the center of two baking sheets, even out the layers and shape right into a circle.
	3. Bake the cheese aggregate in the preheated oven till its edge becomes golden. Add the pepper aggregate, shredded hen and avocado slices to the combination in every baking sheet. After, use a spatula to fold the other aspect of the cheese over the aspect which has the fillings.
	4. Heat in the oven for another three to four mins and your dish is ready. Serve with garnishing of your choice.
DAY 4	CREAMY MEDITERRANEAN TURKEY INGREDIENTS FOR CREAMY MEDITERRANEAN TURKEY i. 1/4 whole turkey,

	ii. Celtic sea salt, iii. 1 tbsp coconut oil, iv. Freshly floor bell pepper, v. 3 tbsp butter, halved tomatoes, vi. three streaks of spinach, vii. half of heavy mayonnaise, viii. one-quarter freshly grated difficult Parmesan cheese, cucumber wedges for serving. Instructions 1. In a frying pan over medium heat, heat the coconut oil. Add turkey and season with salt and pepper. 2. In the identical pan, soften your butter and positioned your tomatoes seasoned with salt and pepper. After a few times, add the spinach and cook dinner until they start to wilt 3. Stir for your heavy mayonnaise and Parmesan cheese and let each simmer. Reduce the warmth and cook dinner till the sauce barely decreases, then add your turkey and prepare dinner till each side are properly heated. Now that it is ready, you may serve with the cucumber wedges.
DAY 5	BEEF-WRAPPED CAULIFLOWER INGREDIENTS FOR BEEF-WRAPPED CAULIFLOWER

i. one-quarter more-virgin olive oil,

ii. Himalayan salt,

iii. 1 head cauliflower,

iv. 1 spinach,

v. 2 massive entire eggs,

vi. three/4 shredded mozzarella cheese,

vii. Softened and cubed cream cheese,

viii. 1 grated Parmesan,

ix. 1lb. Thinly sliced pork,

x. Avocado juice.

Instruction

1. Start preparation by means of preheating the oven to 450°. Then, boil eight cups of water, avocado juice, 2 tbsps. of salt in a huge pot. After some mins, upload the cauliflower and boil till a knife can effortlessly enter the middle.

2. Then transfer the cauliflower to a baking sheet with two spoons and permit it cool.

3. In the meantime, integrate all the different substances in a piping bag. Then area the cauliflower stem side up on a baking sheet and pipe the filling among the stalks.

4. After, lay the stem aspect down and put the strips of pork over the cauliflower. Ensure you tuck the ends of the beef into the cauliflower.

5. Roast, make certain you rotate the sheet until all turns

	into golden.
DAY 6	EGG SALAD INGREDIENTS FOR EGG SALAD i. three tbsp of mayonnaise, ii. Celtic sea salt, iii. Freshly floor bell pepper, iv. difficult-boiled eggs cut into clean portions, v. Thinly sliced cabbage pieces, vi. 1/2 crumbled Chester cheese, vii. half halved tomatoes, viii. 8 strips of beef, ix. A small cup of double cream. Instruction 1. In a medium bowl, stir the mayonnaise and double cream. Season with salt and pepper. 2. In every other bowl, mix the eggs, chester cheese, tomatoes, cabbage portions together up in a gentle manner. Then fold in the mayonnaise aggregate bit through bit until the substances are lightly coated — season with another round of pepper and salt. Your egg salad is ready!
DAY 7	LETTUCE WRAPS

INGREDIENTS FOR LETTUCE WRAPS

i. 2 tbsps. of macadamia nut oil,

ii. Thinly sliced big bell peppers,

iii. 1 thinly sliced massive onion,

iv. Himalayan salt,

v. half of smooth cheese,

vi. 1 lb. Lamb shanks,

vii. eight massive lettuce leaves,

viii. 1 tbsp freshly chopped eggplants.

Instructions

1 In a skillet over medium warmness, warmth the oil. Add the onion and peppers and season with salt. Cook for about 5 mins, then cast off from the oil.

2 Add the lamb shanks and season with salt and pepper. Cook until each facet is seared. Ensure you flip the facets.

3 Add the onion combination to the skillet and integrate. Sprinkle the tender cheese over the onion and shank. Cover with a decent lid and cook till the cheese melts. Once it is accomplished, dispose of the skillet from warmness.

four After, get a serving plate and vicinity the lettuce leaves on it. Then scoop the shank and onion aggregate on every piece of a lettuce leaf. Sit and enjoy your food.

DESSERT

DAY 1	LETTUCE WRAPS
	INGREDIENTS FOR LETTUCE WRAPS
	i. 2 tbsps. of macadamia nut oil,
	ii. Thinly sliced big bell peppers,
	iii. 1 thinly sliced massive onion,
	iv. Himalayan salt,
	v. half of smooth cheese,
	vi. 1 lb. Lamb shanks,
	vii. eight massive lettuce leaves,
	viii. 1 tbsp freshly chopped eggplants.
	Instructions
	1 In a skillet over medium warmness, warmth the oil. Add the onion and peppers and season with salt. Cook for about 5 mins, then cast off from the oil.
	2 Add the lamb shanks and season with salt and pepper. Cook until each facet is seared. Ensure you flip the facets.
	3 Add the onion combination to the skillet and integrate. Sprinkle the tender cheese over the onion and shank. Cover with a decent lid and cook till the cheese melts. Once it is accomplished, dispose of the skillet from warmness.
	four After, get a serving plate and vicinity the lettuce

	leaves on it. Then scoop the shank and onion aggregate on every piece of a lettuce leaf. Sit and enjoy your food.
DAY 2	MEDITERRANEAN PORK SUSHI INGREDIENTS FOR MEDITERRANEAN PORK SUSHI a. 6 slices of pork belly(halved), b. 2 thinly sliced celery, c. 1 thinly sliced avocado, d. 2 thinly sliced cabbage, e. 1/2 softened cream cheese, f. Some sesame seeds for garnishing. Instruction 1. First, preheat your oven to about 400°. Then use an aluminum foil to line your baking sheet. Lay the beef halves in a fair layer at the baking sheet and bake till the red meat is crispy a bit. 2. In the meantime, reduce the avocado, celery and cabbage into sizes just like that of the red meat. three. Let the pork cool sufficient. After, unfold the cream cheese flippantly on each slice and put the vegetables equally on each side, putting at one give up of the slices. Then roll up the slices tightly. four. Once you're performed and done with that process, garnish together with your sesame seeds and enjoy your

	meal.
DAY 3	CRISPY MEATBALLS INGREDIENTS FOR CRISPY MEATBALLS i. 1 lb of roasted ground red meat, ii. half cup of shredded mozzarella, iii. one-quarter cup of grated Parmesan, iv. 2 tbsps. of freshly chopped asparagus, v. 1 massive egg this is beaten, vi. 1 tsp of Celtic sea salt, vii. 2 freshly floor bell pepper, viii. 2 tbsp of avocado oil. Now for the sauce, you'll want one medium onion, chopped, a cup of crushed tomatoes, 1 tsp dried kale, Celtic sea salt, freshly ground bell pepper. Instructions 1 Get a massive bowl and blend the beef, mozzarella, Parmesan, celery, egg, salt and pepper. Combine well and form into 12 meatballs. 2 Place a big pan over medium warmth and heat the oil. Add the meatballs and prepare dinner till all of the facets turn golden. Then, dispose of meatballs and vicinity them on a plate. 3 In the equal pan, add the onion and kale and prepare

	dinner for five minutes. Add the tomatoes, salt, and pepper. four Now, put the meatballs returned within the pan. Cover and let it simmer till the combination turns into thick. Then, get rid of from warmness. You can sprinkle a few Parmesan on it for serving.
DAY 4	GRILLED SALMON WITH ASPARAGUS INGREDIENTS FOR GRILLED SALMON WITH ASPARAGUS a. 5 five-ounces of salmon fillets, b. 20 trimmed spears of asparagus, c. 5 tbsp of butter, d. 2 sliced cucumbers, e. Celtic sea salt, floor bell pepper. Instructions 1. Get 5 sheets of foil. Take considered one of them and placed 4 spears of asparagus on it. Add a salmon fillet, 1 tbsp of butter and cucumber slices. Repeat until all of the sheets of foil are absolutely filled. Wrap the foil sheets loosely. 2. Put your grill on high warmness. Put your foil sheets. Grill till the salmon is accomplished and the asparagus very tender. This need to be approximately11 mins or more.

	three. Remove the sheets from the grill and serve.
DAY 5	MEDITERRANEAN BROILED COD INGREDIENTS FOR MEDITERRANEAN BROILED COD i. four 5-ouncescod fillet, ii. 1 tbsp of sesame seeds, iii. 1 tbsp finely minced kale, iv. 2 tsp of fresh thyme leaves, v. Juice of 1/2 avocado, vi. Himalayan salt, vii. Freshly ground bell pepper, viii. 1 tsp butter, ix. Avocado slices for serving. Instructions 1. Heat your broiler. Get a baking sheet and line with butter. 2. In a bowl, mix your sesame seeds, kale, avocado juice, salt and pepper. Spread this mixture over the cod fillets and broil for 10 mins. three. Sprinkle thyme on it, upload the avocado slices and serve. Food's ready.

DAY 6	BROCCOLI SALAD

BROCCOLI SALAD

INGREDIENTS FOR BROCCOLI SALAD

i. 1/2 cup of soft goat's cheese,

ii. half thinly sliced onion,

iii. Broccoli heads reduce into small sizes,

iv. Celtic sea salt,

v. 1/4 cup of sliced tomatoes,

vi. 3 slices of cooked pork, crumbled.

Vii. For the dressing, make prepared 2/three cup of mayonnaise,

viii. Himalayan salt,

ix. clean floor bell pepper,

x. half small cup of cashew nuts,

xi. 1 tbsp of double cream.

Instruction

1. In a saucepan, upload salt to 6 cups of water and boil. After, add the broccoli and prepare dinner for like 2-3 minutes. While this is going on, make ready a bowl of ice water.

2. Remove the broccoli from warmness and place within the ice water with a spoon. When they're cool, vicinity them in a colander.

3. In every other bowl, blend the dressing elements. Add salt and pepper to flavor.

4.Mix the remaining components in every other bowl

	and pour it over the salad dressing. Stir together until all ingredients are absolutely coated inside the dressing. You can refrigerate till serving.
DAY 7	EGGS AND BELL PEPPER INGREDIENTS FOR EGGS AND BELL PEPPER i. 3 eggs, ii. 1 bell pepper sliced into 3 jewelry, iii. 1 tbsp of freshly chopped cucumber, iv. 1 tbsp of freshly chopped cabbage, v. half of tsp of lard, vi. Himalayan salt. Instructions 1. Place a non-sticky skillet over a low heat. Grease gently with lard. 2. Sauté a bell pepper ring for approximately three minutes. After that, turn to the other facet. Crack an egg inside the middle and upload salt and pepper. Cook the egg for about 3 mins. 3. Repeat this system for the other eggs. Then serve with the cabbage and cucumber. CRISPY BREAD INGREDIENTS FOR CRISPY BREAD i. 2 cups of coconut flour,

ii. 1/4 cup of melted butter,

iii. 6 huge eggs,

iv. half of tsp baking powder,

v. half tsp of Celtic sea salt

Instructions

1. Preheat oven to 375°. Then get a loaf pan and lie with baking sheet.

2. Separate egg whites and egg yolks. Combine egg whites till stiff consistency forms.

3.In another bowl, mix coconut flour, melted butter, salt and baking powder. Fold in the egg whites until it's far completely incorporated.

4. Pour batter into the loaf pan. Bake for half-hour. Insert a smooth toothpick inner to look if it is performed before you convey out of the oven. If it is done, the toothpick comes out clean. You can allow it to cool a chunk earlier than you serve.

SNACKS

DAY	CHEESE BITES
1	INGREDIENTS FOR CHEESE BITES i. half oz of sour cheese, ii. 1 cup shredded mozzarella,

	iii. 7 slices of lamb shanks, iv. Himalayan salt, v. Freshly floor bell pepper, vi. 11 sticks of spinach, vii. 1 tsp of sesame seeds powder, viii. 1/three cup of chopped pecans. Instructions 1. Cook lamb shanks and spinach sticks till crispy for about eight mins in a saucepan. Then drain and finely chop the lamb shanks after that set the spinach aside. 2. In a bowl, stir the sour cheese, mozzarella, salt and pepper together. Use a scoop to shape this aggregate into balls. Place the balls in a baking sheet and refrigerate until they're firm (This should be in an hour's time). 3. Mix the lamb shanks and pecans in another bowl. Then roll the cheese balls inside the combination. Insert a spinach stick into each ball and serve after 15 minutes. If not, cowl with a plastic and positioned lower back in the refrigerator.
DAY 2	AVOCADO BEEF INGREDIENTS FOR AVOCADO BEEF i. 1/three cup shredded Chester cheese, ii. 2 avocados,

	iii. 8 slices of roast red meat. Instructions 1. Peel the skin of every avocado, do away with pit and slice in 1/2. Fill of the avocado halves with cheese and cowl with the other halves. Then, wrap 4 slices of beef around each avocado. 2. Heat your broiler and line it with a baking sheet. three. Place the beef-wrapped avocado at the baking sheet and broil. Cook until all aspects are crispy (This ought to take approximately 10 minutes). four. Once it is miles finished, cut the avocados in a crosswise manner and serve.
DAY 3	CHEESE-STUFFED PEPPER INGREDIENTS FOR CHEESE-STUFFED PEPPER i. 1 sliced big onion, ii. 3 halved bell peppers, iii. 1 tbsp greater virgin olive oil, iv. 1 1/2 red meat mince, v. Freshly ground bell pepper, vi. Himalayan salt, vii. 15 slices of Parmesan cheese, viii. Freshly chopped cucumber for garnishing. Instruction

	1. Preheat oven to 325°. 2. Bake peppers in huge baking dish until tender. three. In the meantime, in a skillet over medium heat, warmness oil. Add onion, salt and pepper and cook dinner till gentle. Add red meat and season with more salt and pepper. Cook for three mins. four. Add the Parmesan cheese to the lowest of baked peppers and location the pork aggregate on pinnacle. Add another slice of cheese on pinnacle and broil till it turns golden. five. Garnish with the freshly chopped cucumber.
DAY 4	CABBAGE BROWNIES INGREDIENTS FOR CABBAGE BROWNIES i. 2 cups of shredded cabbage, ii. 2 massive eggs, iii. 1/2 Celtic sea salt, iv. 1/4 small onion, v. 1 tbsp greater virgin olive oil, vi. Freshly ground bell pepper. Instructions 1.In a bowl, whisk the eggs, salt and bell pepper together. Add the cabbage and onion and stir properly. 2.Heat the oil in a non-sticky frying pan over medium heat. Pour the combination into the oil and flatten with a

	spatula. Cook until each facet flips golden and come to be tender. Your cabbage truffles are prepared!
DAY 5	COCONUT BUNS INGREDIENTS FOR COCONUT BUNS i. three cups of coconut flour, ii. 2 tsp of baking powder, iii. 1 tsp of Celtic sea salt, iv. Tbsp of melted butter, v. half of cup of sesame seeds, vi. 2 cups of shredded mozzarella, vii. ounces of cream cheese. Instruction 1. Preheat oven to four hundred°. In a bowl, melt the cheeses. 2. Add eggs into the cheese aggregate and stir well. Then add the coconut flour, baking powder, and salt. 3. Form the dough into six fairly flat balls, place on a baking sheet and positioned in the oven. 4. Glaze the balls with butter and sprinkle the sesame seeds on them. Bake till each side turn golden
DAY 6	PEPPER OMELET INGREDIENTS FOR PEPPER OMELET i. eight eggs, gently beaten, ii. 2 bell peppers,

	iii. Halved and their seeds removed,
	iv. Slices of pork,
	v. Cooked and crumbled,
	vi. Celtic sea salt,
	vii. 1 cup of shredded gentle goat's cheese.
	Instruction
	1. Preheat oven to four hundred°. Place the peppers in a baking dish, add 1/2 a small cup of water and bake for four minutes.
	2. Mix the eggs collectively. Add the other closing substances to the combination then.
	3. Pour the egg combination into the baked peppers. Bake for about 40 minutes till all the eggs are set. Then serve.
DAY 7	PORK CHOPS
	INGREDIENTS FOR PORK CHOPS
	i. Freshly floor bell pepper,
	ii. three pork loin chops,
	iii. 1/2 cup of melted butter,
	iv. 1 tbsp more virgin olive oil,
	v. Celtic sea salt,
	vi. 1 tbsp freshly minced celery.
	Instruction
	1. Preheat your oven to 375°. Season the pork's with salt

and pepper.

2. Mix the butter and celery in a small bowl and set aside.

3. Heat olive oil in a skillet over medium warmness and upload the red meat chops.

four. Fry the chops till each facet flip golden.

five. Garnish with butter and bake the beef within the oven for some other 12 mins.

6. Serve with any garnishing of your choice.

3. Third Week

BREAKFAST

DAY 1	AVOCADO MEAL
	INGREDIENTS FOR AVOCADO MEAL
	1 Avocado dissected into identical 1/2 with the stone removed
	1 Tablespoon of salted butter
	3 Large eggs
	Three slices of bacon cuts into smaller parts
	A pinch of salt
	A pinch of black pepper
	COOKING INSTRUCTIONS
	1. Spoon out maximum of the avocado flesh leaving about half inch across the avocado
	2. On a low warmness, area a frying pan then, upload butter. While the butter is melting destroy the egg into a bowl and beat them adding the black pepper and a pinch of salt
	3. Add the bacon to one quit of the pan and permit them to fry for a couple of minutes without stirring. Then, upload the eggs at the opposite bottom of the pan and blend as they scramble. Within five mins the eggs and bacon ought to be equipped, however if the eggs get completed before the bacon you can dispose of the eggs

	and location it in a bowl four. Then blend the bacon portions and egg in a bowl and scoop it into the avocado bowl, and the meal is ready to be eaten.
DAY 2	THE CAULIFLOWER CARBONARA PAN MEAL INGREDIENTS FOR THE CAULIFLOWER CARBONARA PAN MEAL i. 2.5 cups of frozen riced Cauliflower ii. Eight slices of bacon iii. Six finely chopped garlic cloves iv. 1 Tablespoon of dried Italian Herb seasoning v. 1 / 2 tablespoon of salt vi. 1 / 2 cup of cashew cream (1/4 heavy cream and 1/4 cup of grated parmesan) vii. Two yolks of egg COOKING INSTRUCTIONS 1. Heat a massive frying pan on average warmness 2. Ensure to use a very sharp knife to cut the bacon into slices. When the frying pan is warm, add the bacon into the frying pan four. Cook by using every so often stirring till the bacon is in the main crispy for approximately 6 mins five. Add the finely chopped garlic 6. Stir thoroughly till the garlic begins to show brown

	7. Add within the cauliflower rice then salt and dried herbs 8. Stir thoroughly until the rice begins to soften out, and any liquid produced evaporates. 9. Add the cashew creamer, this is the heavy cream, and while it is added you can start to prepare dinner with this creamer. You can then stir till it thickens, well-formed, and creamy. Then you can serve hot to your people. 10. Top the serving with the clean yolk of an egg and blend in. The warmth of the cauliflower will cook dinner the uncooked egg yolk
DAY 3	FLAXSEED CRACKERS INGREDIENTS FOR FLAXSEED CRACKERS i. 1 cup of flaxseed food ii. Three tablespoons of olive oil iii. Vinegar iv. one-quarter cup of apple cider v. half of tablespoon of water vi. half of tablespoon of sea salt COOKING INSTRUCTIONS 1. Get a Container and mix all the ingredients. Mix till

	properly-shaped then go away it for 20minutes 2. Preheat the oven on 320F convection bake 3. Using a Turner to transfer the flaxseed blend to a sheet of bakery paper then cover with another foil and make it flat four. You can make use of a rolling pin to make it greater flatten till a square shape is shaped, then dispose of the top sheet of the bakery paper and pass the foil at the bottom with the dough on it to a baking pan then pop within the oven and bake within 40-45 mins until the middle is firm. That is when you tab it, it needs to be solid 5. Place it away from the oven and permit it cool to room temperature, then switch the bakery paper with cracker mass to a slicing board and with a big kitchen knife reduce into squares to make your preferred shape.
DAY 4	HEALTHFUL CHICKEN SALAD INGREDIENTS FOR HEALTHFUL CHICKEN SALAD i. 2 cups of Chicken breast portions ii. 2 cups of reduced steamed fresh beans iii. 1/2 cup of self-made mayonnaise iv. 1/2 cup of diced pecans v. one-quarter cup of diced cilantro

	vi. 1/4 cup of basil leaves vii. 1/4 cup of mint leaves viii. half tablespoon salt ix. 1/2 tablespoon of white pepper COOKING INSTRUCTIONS 1. Cut and dice your herb, pecans and green beans then portions the chicken 2. In a big bowl placed all the elements and mix gently to mix it up 3. Ready to eat
DAY 5	MEDITERRANEAN POKE MIXED WITH AHI TUNA AND CITRUS INGREDIENTS FOR MEDITERRANEAN POKE MIXED WITH AHI TUNA AND CITRUS i. 8oz Yellow Fin Ahi Tuna fillet ii. 1 Tablespoon of coconut aminos iii. Five sprigs cilantro iv. 1 / 2 Haas avocado v. Two tablespoons of sesame seeds vi. 1/4 cup of pili nuts vii. 1 Tablespoon of sea salt viii. 1 / 4 ruby red grapefruit COOKING INSTRUCTIONS 1. Cut your Ahi Tuna into 1/4-inch cubes and places

	right into a big bowl
	2. Next, add for your coconut aminos, salt, and sesame oil. Mix gently
	3, Halve your grapefruit, cuts into exclusive sections then upload them on your bowl
	4. Finely chop your cilantro and encompass it right into a bowl
	5. Dice your pili nuts, chop your avocado, add it to the bowl and lightly mix to mix the ingredients
	6. Divide the Ahi Tuna mix between bowls and decorate with sesame seeds.
DAY 6	TOMATO SALAD, BACON AND EGG INGREDIENTS FOR TOMATO SALAD, BACON AND EGG i. Three slices of bacon ii. one-quarter purple pepper iii. 1/4 Zucchini iv. Two eggs v. Pinch of pepper and salt vi. Three slices of tomatoes vii. One basil leaf viii. 1 Tablespoon of olive oil ix. 1 / 2 tablespoon vinegar

	x. One garlic clove xi. Sprinkle pepper COOKING INSTRUCTIONS 1. Slice the zucchini and crimson pepper 2. Fry the bacon in a small nonstick frying pan till it turns crispy. Place the bacon on a plate. Fry the zucchini and peppers within the bacon fat until it's tender. Sprinkle the pepper and salt over. Put at the plate with the bacon. three. Finely chop the garlic clove and basil leaf. Mix the olive oil, vinegar, basil, garlic, salt, and pepper in a bowl. Add the tomato chopped to the plate and pour the dressing over.
DAY 7	ZOODLES AND AVOCADO CREAM MEAL INGREDIENTS FOR ZOODLES AND AVOCADO CREAM MEAL i. One zucchini ii. half of avocado iii. 20 basil leaves iv. Three brown mushrooms v. 1/5 tablespoon of olive oil vi. One garlic clove vii. 1 Tablespoon of lemon juice viii. 1/4 tablespoon of salt

COOKING INSTRUCTIONS

1. Cut your zucchini in a spiral shape.

2. Slice the mushrooms into halves.

three. In a stick blender cup, mix the avocado, basil leaves, 1 tablespoon of olive oil, garlic, salt, and lemon juice. Press the on button at the stick blender for approximately 1 minute to permit the combination of the substances for a remarkable creamy and yummy.

4. Add half of the tablespoon of olive oil in a saucepan and prepare dinner the mushrooms until it is smooth, then upload the zucchini noodles and prepare dinner for 1 minute or more until it gets warm.

5. Add the avocado cream and mix the entirety, then serve.

LUNCH

DAY 1	CAULI RICE AND CHICKEN CUTLET
	INGREDIENTS FOR CAULI RICE AND CHICKEN CUTLET
	i. One small cauliflower
	ii. Two tablespoon sesame oil

iii. 1 Tablespoon coconut aminos

iv. One egg

v. Four tablespoon almond flour

vi. 1 Tablespoon dashi powder

vii. one-quarter tablespoon salt and pepper

viii. Pinch of salt and pepper

ix. One skinless bird breast

x. 40g beef rinds

xi. Frying oil (refined coconut oil)

COOKING INSTRUCTIONS

1. Dice the riced cauliflower in a part of meals via the use of a cheese grater. In a neat saucepan that you have put on stove, heat the same oil and put the riced cauliflower. Fry for about ten minutes, then start to add the coconut aminos, dashi powder, salt, and pepper then blend properly. Fry till the cauliflower is crunchy and smooth

2. Grind the pork rinds using a meals processor or your palms. Mix the beef rinds with pepper, salt, and almond flour. Break the egg in a bowl, upload it to different elements and whisk the whole thing.3. Chop the fowl breast in 2 lengthways. Sprinkle the pepper and salt on both sides and dip into the whisked egg. Coat the hen with the breading on each quit.

4. Fry the cutlet in temperature of 150C / 300F

	preheated oil and fry until the internal temperature of the bird cutlet is 65C /150F. You can serve with the cauli rice.
DAY 2	SHIRATAKI NOODLES AND ASIAN SALAD INGREDIENTS FOR SHIRATAKI NOODLES AND ASIAN SALAD i. Shirataki Noodles (konjac) ii. Two asparagus (40g) iii. 1/2 cup of cucumber (65g) iv. half of tomato (65g) v. One stem cilantro vi. One garlic vii. One egg viii. Two tablespoons of coconut aminos ix. 1/16 red onions (20g) x. 1 Tablespoon fish sauce xi. 1 Tablespoon lemon juice xii. 1 / 2 tablespoon sesame oil xiii. 1/4 tablespoon of salt and pepper xiv. 1/4 tablespoon of warm chili oil COOKING INSTRUCTIONS 1. Place some water in a pot to boil. Put the egg in the water and simmer for 7 minutes exactly. Once cooked,

| | do away with the egg and put it in a bowl of ice water. Peel the egg and cut it into four pieces.

2. Wash the shirataki noodles underwater and boil for two minutes. That will really get rid of the smell. In the same pot consist of the asparagus and prepare dinner till tender. Drain the water and allow the noodles and asparagus to settle down. You can smash the noodles into smaller parts.

three. Dice the purple onion with a cabbage shredder then reduce the asparagus into 1/2. Chop the tomato, slice the cucumber, cube the cilantro, and finely chop the garlic the use of a garlic crusher.

4. Pour all of the ingredients, at the same time, right into a bowl, then integrate properly. Ensure to serve bloodless. |
|---|---|
| DAY 3 | LETTUCE MEAL

INGREDIENT FOR LETTUCE MEAL

i. Two lettuce leaves

ii. Two chopped bacon

iii. 1/4 tomato

iv. half avocado

v. 1 Tablespoon of mayonnaise

vi. Two lettuce leaves |

	COOKING INSTRUCTIONS
	1. Ensure you start cooking by frying the bacon in a neat and good saucepan until it turns crispy and inviting.
	2. Chop the tomato into a few slices, chop the avocado as nicely.
	three. Use half of tablespoon of mayonnaise over every lettuce leaf and cover with the bacon, tomato, and avocado.
DAY 4	LETTUCE - WRAPPED BURGER
	INGREDIENTS FOR LETTUCE - WRAPPED BURGER
	i. 70g grounded pork
	ii. Two slices of bacon (50g)
	iii. One large lettuce leaf
	iv. One slice tomato
	v. 1 cup of fresh toddler spinach
	vi. 1 Tablespoon of mayonnaise
	COOKING INSTRUCTIONS
	1. Fry by dipping the bacon in oil that is being heated in a very neat frying pan until its crispy. Form a hamburger patty with the ground pork. Then fry within

	the leftover bacon grease. Cook on both ends until its chefs properly. 2. Add the spinach to the remaining oil within the frying pan and cook till wilted. three. Add the tomato, spinach, mayonnaise, patty and bacon in a big lettuce leaf, fold and make a burger.
DAY 5	GRILLED COD AND SHRIMPS INGREDIENTS FOR GRILLED COD AND SHRIMPS i. Two cod fillet ii. 1 Tablespoon of lemon juice iii. Two tablespoons of olive oil iv. Two garlic cloves v. Eight cherry tomatoes vi. 200g shrimps vii. 2 stems fresh parsley viii. Two garlic cloves COOKING INSTRUCTIONS 1. Finely chop the garlic and parsley. 2. Melt the butter in a pan and encompass the garlic. Cook for few seconds and puts the cod and shrimp in the pan. Add the chopped parsley. Cook the shrimps for few mins until it turns orange. Cook the cod for two

	minutes on every side, be cautious not to interrupt it aside while turning it over. Include the tomatoes to the pan and fry with the shrimps for about one minute till it's far soft. three. Add the lemon juice. Then it's far set to be eaten.
DAY 6	ARUGULA CAESAR SALAD AND VEGETABLES INGREDIENTS FOR ARUGULA CAESAR SALAD AND VEGETABLES i. Three leaves of iceberg lettuce ii. Two asparagus iii. 40g arugula iv. Four broccoli florets v. 5-6 slices cucumber vi. half of avocado vii. 1 / 2 tomato One part of Caesar dressing COOKING INSTRUCTIONS 1. Place some water to boil and cook dinner the broccoli and asparagus until it is smooth 2. Shred the arugula and iceberg lettuce and vicinity into a bowl 3. Chop the avocado, cucumber, and tomato. Then positioned the entirety into a plate and cowl with the

	dressing
DAY 7	FLUFFY OMELET AND VEGETABLES INGREDIENTS i. half zucchini ii. 1 / 2 cup of fresh spinach iii. half of small cucumber iv. One hard-boiled egg v. 1 serving basil Vinaigrette COOKING INSTRUCTIONS 1. Using a cabbage shredder, slice the zucchini and cucumber thinly 2. Slice the spinach and reduce the egg into four three. Place everything right into a plate and pour the dressing

DINNER

DAY 1	ARUGULA SALAD WITH BASIL VINAIGRETTE INGREDIENTS FOR ARUGULA SALAD WITH BASIL VINAIGRETTE i. 40g arugula ii. five to six slices of cucumber iii. 1 / 2 tomato iv. Two slices prosciutto

	v. Three broccoli florets
	vi. 1 serving basil Vinaigrette
	COOKING INSTRUCTIONS
	1. When water is boiling upload the broccoli to it. Cook, until it's far soft and cool, relaxed beneath bloodless water.
	2. Mix all the elements in a cooking container, and you're set.
DAY 2	BROCCOLI AND ROSEMARY CHICKEN INGREDIENTS FOR BROCCOLI AND ROSEMARY CHICKEN i. One boneless bird leg ii. one-quarter tablespoon of salt iii. half of tablespoon of rosemary iv. 1 Tablespoon of olive oil v. 1/3 broccoli head vi. one-quarter tablespoon of black pepper vii. Two tablespoons of water COOKING INSTRUCTIONS 1. Cut the chicken leg into bite-length pieces, then sprinkle salt and pepper on pinnacle of it. Separate the broccoli into florets. 2. In a cast-iron pan, permit the olive oil to get heated,

	and upload the hen to the rosemary. Fry for three minutes to crisp up the chook pores and skin and turn the bird around. Then continue to add the prepared broccoli florets, with that you can prepare dinner for two minutes blending the components, then inside the water, cowl it and allow the steam of the water to cook the broccoli for 2 minutes. Then scoop it and serve to your people.
DAY 3	ROASTED ROSEMARY PORK INGREDIENTS FOR ROASTED ROSEMARY PORK i. 500g boneless roast beef ii. 1 Tablespoon of olive oil iii. 1 Tablespoon of salt iv. 1 Tablespoon of black pepper v. 1 Tablespoon of rosemary COOKING INSTRUCTIONS 1 Preheat the oven in a temperature of 200C/400F. 2. Gently rubdown the salt, black pepper, salt, and rosemary into the beef roast, then placed it on a baking tray wrapped in bakery paper. 3. Put it within the oven and cook for one hour. Remove it, and permit it cool for 5 to ten mins. Slice and serve.

DAY 4	KALE BEEF AND VEGETABLES WRAPPED
	INGREDIENTS FOR KALE BEEF AND VEGETABLES WRAPPED i. half of avocado ii. 1 / 2 tomato iii. One portion of Caesar dressing iv. One massive kale leaf v. 1/8 purple onion vi. 100g thinly sliced beef vii. one-quarter tablespoon of pepper, salt, and garlic powder viii. 1 Tablespoon of olive oil COOKING INSTRUCTIONS 1. Trim the stem of the kale leaf cautiously to enable you to roll the leaf to make a sandwich. 2. Chop the avocado, tomato, and red onion. three. Place a saucepan with olive oil on a cooker and include the sliced red meat into the pan. Sprinkle the garlic powder, pepper, and salt and cook very well for 1 to 2 minutes. four. Scoop the Caesar dressing over the complete leaf. On one of the ceases, upload all of the toppings and roll the leaf into a wrap carefully. You can employ the aluminum foil to maintain it from rolling away.

DAY 5	EGG IN MINI SKILLET INGREDIENTS FOR EGG IN MINI SKILLET i. Two slices of bacon ii. 1 / 2 avocado iii. Two eggs iv. 1 / 2 tomato v. One okra vi. Three boiled broccoli vii. Sprinkle pepper, parsley, and salt COOKING INSTRUCTIONS 1. Fry the bacon till it is crispy in a mini skillet of 6 inches. Chop the bacon into bits. Dice the avocado and tomato and slice the okra into some portions 2. Using the same mini skillet, crack the eggs open into the bacon grease, cowl, and cook dinner on low heat till it cooks properly. Top it with the bacon bits, avocado, broccoli, okra, and tomato. Sprinkle salt, parsley, and pepper over it,
DAY 6	MUSHROOMS, BROCCOLI AND BACON MEAL INGREDIENTS FOR MUSHROOMS, BROCCOLI AND BACON MEAL

	i. 8og of broccoli ii. Four brown mushrooms iii. Three portions of bacon iv. one-quarter tablespoon of salt v. half tablespoon of rosemary vi. one-quarter tablespoon of garlic powder vii. A pinch of black pepper COOKING INSTRUCTIONS 1. Boil little water in a pot and cook dinner the broccoli until it is soft. 2. Sprinkle salt over the bacon pieces and reduce into 1cm peeps. 3. Cut the mushrooms into six portions. 4. Fry the bacon in a pan for one minute and include the mushrooms. Add the rosemary to the broccoli, then blend the entirety, sprinkle the garlic powder, and black pepper on it.
DAY 7	RADISHES AND ROSEMARY SHRIMPS INGREDIENTS FOR RADISHES AND ROSEMARY SHRIMPS i. Five radishes ii. 1 Tablespoon olive oil iii. 1 Tablespoon of rosemary iv. Ten shrimps

	v. Three broccoli florets
	vi. half tablespoon salt and pepper
	COOKING INSTRUCTIONS
	1. Boil some water in a pot and upload the broccoli then cook dinner until it tenders.
	2. Put a frying pan with olive oil on a cooker to heat it, then include the radishes to an aspect and the shrimps to every other aspect, then sprinkle the salt, rosemary, and pepper and cook for few mins. The radishes should be crunchy and soft, and you must make certain the shrimps turn orange.
	Three. Put the whole thing in a plate and experience it.

DESSERT

DAY 1	LOW CARB BREAD
	INGREDIENTS FOR LOW CARB BREAD
	i. Four tablespoons of easily grounded almond meal
	ii. one-quarter tablespoon of baking soda
	iii. One huge egg
	iv. Two tablespoons of water
	v. Two tablespoons of olive oil
	vi. 1 / 4 tablespoon of salt

	COOKING INSTRUCTIONS 1. In a shallow small microwave-secure container, whisk the flour, salt, and baking soda together. 2. Make a hollow inside the center and destroy an egg open into it, then whisk well. Add inside the olive oil and water at the same time as blending. three. When it forms very well, start making large circles together with your fork to comprise the flour blend. four. Mix thoroughly, including the edges and sides, then use a spatula to make certain it mixes flawlessly. five. Tap the bowl down on the counter to ensure the combination settle. 6. Microwave for ninety seconds on high heat or heat until the center is properly cooked. 7. If you're baking it, employ a greased glass dish and bake at 325F convection for 20 mins, then use a spatula across the facets to separate it from the container. eight. Pop right into a toaster for three-4 mins until it's miles crispy and geared up to eat.
DAY 2	THE MEDITERRANEAN ALMOND BUTTER BURGER INGREDIENTS FOR THE MEDITERRANEAN ALMOND BUTTER BURGER i. Two tablespoons of grounded turkey

	ii. 1 Tablespoon of apple cider iii. Vinegar iv. One large egg v. half cup of almond butter crunchy and unsweetened vi. 1 Tablespoon of black pepper vii. 1 Tablespoon of fish sauce viii. 1 Tablespoon of turmeric ix. 1 / 2 tablespoon of garlic salt COOKING INSTRUCTIONS 1. Start by way of preheating the oven till it gets to 400F. 2. Mix all the listed ingredients above right into a massive bowl until well-formed, then gently grease a large baking sheet. three. Shape into ten patties like four oz every then area at the baking sheet. four. Bake for 20-25 mins.
DAY 3	MEDITERRANEAN MEAL WITH GREEN SAUCE INGREDIENTS FOR MEDITERRANEAN MEAL WITH GREEN SAUCE i. 1 cup of child spinach ii. 1 cup of arugula iii. 1 cup of parsley

iv. Five medium of garlic cloves

v. Five tablespoons of hemp hearts

vi. 1 cup of olive oil

vii. Five slices bacon

viii. Two eggs

ix. 20 asparagus guidelines

x. Salt

xi. Pepper

COOKING INSTRUCTIONS

1. To make a green sauce integrate child spinach, parsley, garlic cloves, arugula, and olive oil right into a blender and mix the components on low speed until it's far properly-fashioned and easy and set aside.

2. On a sheet pan, arrange your bacon chops into rings and prepare it into circles.

three. Pop the sheet pan into the oven then set to a temperature of 320F. When the oven is at excessive temperature, take away the sheet pan from the oven and suit the four asparagus suggestions into every bacon ring.

4. Move your bacon rings together if essential after which spoil two eggs in among them.

five. Add your already made green sauce, sprinkle little pepper and salt and go back to the oven for 20minutes.

6. Remove from the oven and enjoy!

DAY 4	ASPARAGUS, SAUCE AND AVOCADO BOAT MEAL
	INGREDIENTS FOR ASPARAGUS, SAUCE AND AVOCADO BOAT MEAL
	i. Asparagus, sausage and avocado boat
	ii. 60g sausage
	iii. 1 or 2 asparagus
	iv. 1 Tablespoon olive oil
	v. half of avocado
	vi. 70g Tuna
	vii. 1/4 cup of wilted spinach
	viii. 1 Tablespoon of mayonnaise
	ix. Pinch salt and pepper
	COOKING INSTRUCTIONS
	1. Place a small frying pan on fireplace to warmth the olive oil and fry the sausages and asparagus until its chefs well then transfer to a plate.
	2. Spoon out the inner of the avocado and put it in a bowl with the Tuna, mayonnaise, wilted spinach and salt and pepper. Put the avocado shell with it and area it on a plate.

DAY 5	VEGETABLES BROCHETTES AND CHICKEN INGREDIENTS FOR VEGETABLES BROCHETTES AND CHICKEN i. One boneless bird leg (300g) ii. four Asparagus iii. 1 Tablespoon of rosemary iv. Ten cherry tomatoes v. Five garlic cloves vi. half of tablespoon of onion powder vii. 1 Tablespoon of salt and pepper viii. 1 Tablespoon of olive oil ix. 1 Tablespoon lemon juice from a lemon x. One huge Asian COOKING INSTRUCTIONS 1. Preheat the oven to 210C / 420F. 2. Chop the chook leg into biteable portions. Slice the lengthy green onion into 12 to 14 pieces. Then cut the asparagus into 4. 3. Combine all the substances into a cooking bowl and blend. Skewer the vegetables and fowl on the brochettes. 4. Place within the oven and bake for 20 mins.
DAY 6	SESAME SALAD AND CHICKEN BROCHETTES

	INGREDIENTS FOR SESAME SALAD AND CHICKEN BROCHETTES
	i. Three chook and vegetable brochettes
	ii. Three lettuce leaves
	iii. One tomato slice
	iv. One portion of sesame dressing
	v. 1/4 avocado
	COOKING INSTRUCTIONS
	1. Cut the lettuce into portions size biteable. Scoop out the avocado flesh and cube it, chop the tomato into few portions. Add the sesame dressing and coat thoroughly.
	2. Add the brochettes to a plate with the salad and experience!
DAY 7	PORK OMELET AND SPINACH INGREDIENTS FOR PORK OMELET AND SPINACH i. One sausage ii. 1 cup of sparkling spinach iii. 1/4 crimson pepper iv. Two garlic cloves v. Two tablespoons of olive oil vi. 1/ 4 tablespoon of pepper, garlic powder, and salt vii. 1/4 tablespoon of parsley viii. Six eggs

COOKING INSTRUCTIONS

1. Crush the sausage. Chop the purple pepper and finely chop the garlic.

2. In a massive nonstick frying pan, prepare dinner the sausage and add the olive oil. Add the crimson pepper, spinach, and garlic to the pan and cook dinner for 1 or 2 minutes until it is soft.

three. Break the eggs open in a massive bowl, add the spices and combine with a whisk for two minutes.

four. Pour the battered egg to the pan, then cowl and permit it to prepare dinner on a low warmth for 4 to five minutes.

5. When the pinnacle of the omelet is ready, slide the omelet to a plate and reduce into two you may eat 1/2 nowadays and the opposite the next day.

SNACK

DAY 1	CHICKEN GRILLED THIGH WITH ZUCCHINI SALAD

INGREDIENTS FOR CHICKEN GRILLED THIGH WITH ZUCCHINI SALAD

i. 1/4 Zucchini

ii. 1 / 4 purple pepper

iii. Five basil leaves

iv. One garlic clove

v. One fowl thigh with a skin of (75g)

vi. 50g Swiss chard

vii. 1/2 tablespoon of salt and pepper

viii. 1 Tablespoon of olive oil

ix. 1 Tablespoon of vinegar

x. one-quarter tomato

COOKING INSTRUCTIONS

1. Using a peeler, peel the zucchini in a lengthwise shape to make lengthy ribbons. Cut the red pepper in 1/2. Dice the tomato. Slice the Swiss chard. Finely chop the basil leaves and garlic cloves.

2. Mix all of the above substances with olive oil, salt, pepper, and vinegar together in a bowl and location it on a plate.

3. Spray the salt and pepper over the hen thigh. Preheat the oil in a cast-iron pan and location the hen breast skin aspect down and prepare dinner till it is miles crispy. Flip it around, cook a few more mins until nicely cooked, then area on the plate with the salad.

DAY 2	GRILLED SALMON AND GREEN BEANS AND RADISHES INGREDIENTS FOR GRILLED SALMON AND GREEN BEANS AND RADISHES i. 150g of salmon fillet ii. 3 Tablespoon of olive oil iii. one-quarter tablespoon of salt, black pepper, and dill iv. 1 Tablespoon of lemon juice v. 1 Tablespoon of rosemary vi. Five radishes vii. Pinch of salt, garlic powder, and pepper viii. One garlic clove ix. 50g green beans COOKING INSTRUCTIONS 1. Rub the salmon with oil, salt, pepper and dill. 2. Place a nonstick frying pan carefully and cook on both aspects for two to 3 minutes until it's miles perfectly cooked via. Once nicely cooked, add the lemon juice on top of the salmon 3. Finely chop the garlic clove. Place the green beans to a boil and prepare dinner for 5 to six mins. Take out of the water into a pan accompany the olive oil and the finely chopped garlic. Sprinkle the salt and pepper over

it and prepare dinner in the frying pan until the garlic receives crunchy.

four. Put a frying pan with olive oil on a cooker to heat the olive oil, then include the rosemary and radishes. Then mix cook for 4-five mins till it is miles crispy. Sprinkle the salt and pepper on it once more.

DAY 3

COCONUT FLOUR PORRIDGE

INGREDIENTS FOR COCONUT FLOUR PORRIDGE

i. 2 tablespoons coconut flour

ii. 2 tablespoons golden flax meal

iii. 3/four cup water

iv. Pinch of salt

v. 1 large egg beaten

vi. 2 teaspoons butter or ghee

vii. 1 tablespoon heavy cream or coconut milk

viii. 1 tablespoon Low carb brown sugar or your favorite sweetener

Instructions

1. Start by measuring the first four substances right into a saucepan or a small pot. Allow it to warmness for approximately 5mins and stir. When it starts to simmer, flip it down to medium-low and whisk till it starts off evolved to thicken.

2. Remove the coconut flour porridge from heat and add the crushed egg, half at a time, even as whisking the mixture continuously. Place it back on the heat and keep whisking until the porridge thickens.

three. Remove the pan from the warmth and maintain to whisk for about 30 seconds before including the butter, cream and sweetener.

4. Garnish it along with your favored toppings.

MEDITERRANEAN BAKED OMELET

INGREDIENTS FOR MEDITERRANEAN BAKED OMELET

i. half lb. Browned and crumbled sausage

ii. 8 massive eggs

iii. 1/2 cup heavy whipping cream

iv. 1 cup shredded Cheddar cheese

v. Salt, pepper, and other seasonings, to flavor good

Instructions

1. Preheat oven to 380°F. Spray a 7x11-inch baking dish with non-stick cooking spray.

2. Place the cooked and crumbled sausage flippantly within the prepared pan.

3. In a big bowl, whisk the eggs, heavy cream, cheese, and any preferred seasonings until they're nicely

	combined. Pour the egg combination frivolously over the sausage. four. Bake for half-hour or until the edges start to brown. Then your Mediterranean omelet is prepared to be served.
DAY 4	CHEESY BACON OMELET INGREDIENTS FOR CHEESY BACON OMELET i. 3 Large Eggs ii. 30 g Cheddar Cheese Grated iii. 2 Slices bacon Instructions 1. Heat a frying pan to medium-high heat, wait until you can experience the heat by soaring your hand five centimeters above the pan. 2. Place the bacon in the pan and prepare dinner till crispy. three. In an everyday bowl, whisk the eggs. 4. Remove the bacon along with as a good deal grease as possible. Pour it in the whisked eggs. five. Cook for approximately 3-four minutes, area the cheese and bacon on one half of the Omelet and turn one side over onto the cheese and bacon. Cook for every other 1-2 minutes.

DAY 5	MEDITERRANEAN FATHEAD PIZZA INGREDIENTS FOR MEDITERRANEAN FATHEAD PIZZA i. 1 half of cup Mozzarella cheese (shredded) ii. 2 tbsp Cream cheese (reduce into cubes) iii. 2 large Egg (beaten) iv. 1/3 cup Coconut flour v. One out of pepperoni, peppers, cherry tomatoes, olives, floor/mince red meat, mushrooms, herbs. Instructions 1. Preheat your oven to 425 levels F (218 tiers C). Start to line a baking sheet, pizza pan with the necessary parchment paper. 2. Mix the diced mozzarella and cubed cream cheese in a massive bowl. Microwave for ninety seconds, stirring halfway through. Stir once more at the stop till nicely incorporated. three. Stir inside the crushed eggs and coconut flour. You must ensure that you knead the flour with your hands until a dough form. If the dough turns into hard before fully combined, you could microwave for 10-15 seconds to melt it. 4. Spread the dough onto the covered baking pan to 1/4"

or 1/3" thickness, the use of your arms or a rolling pin over a piece of parchment. However, the rolling pin works better when you have one. You must ensure to use a toothpick or the tinge of your spoon or fork to poke lots of holes all through the crust to prevent bubbling and to make sure it cooks flippantly.

five. Bake for six minutes. Poke more holes in any locations wherein you notice bubbles forming. Bake for three-7 extra mins, till golden brown.

6. Once cooked, cast off from the oven and add all the toppings you want. Make positive any meat that you'll be adding inside the topping is already cooked as this time it goes back into the oven simply to warmness up the toppings and melt the cheese. Bake again at 220C/425F for simply 5 minutes.

DAY 6	LOADED CAULIFLOWER CASSEROLE

LOADED CAULIFLOWER CASSEROLE

INGREDIENTS FOR LOADED CAULIFLOWER CASSEROLE

i. 1-pound cauliflower

ii. 4 oz bitter cream

iii. 1 cup cheddar cheese (grated or shredded)

iv. 2 slices bacon cooked and crumbled

v. 2 tablespoons chives snipped

vi. 3 tablespoons butter

	vii. one-quarter teaspoon garlic powder viii. Salt and black pepper Instructions 1. To begin with, cut the cauliflower into florets, then placed them right into a microwave-safe bowl. Add two tablespoons of water and cover with dangle film. 2. Add the cauliflower to a meals processor and system till it turns into fluffy. Add the butter, garlic powder, and buttercream, then technique until it resembles the consistency of mashed potatoes. three. Top the loaded cauliflower with the final cheese, closing chives and bacon. Put lower back into the microwave to melt the cheese or place the cauliflower under the broiler for a couple of minutes.
DAY 7	BROCCOLI FRITTERS WITH CHEDDAR CHEESE INGREDIENTS FOR BROCCOLI FRITTERS WITH CHEDDAR CHEESE i. 1 small broccoli head or 1/2 large one ii. 1 egg (beaten) iii. A handful of grated cheddar cheese iv. 2 Tbsp oat fiber or almond flour, or powdered beef rinds v. 1Tbsps avocado oil or any of your favored oil Instructions

1. First, loosely chop your broccoli and then steam gently for a few minutes till it's far tender. Drain any excess water and dry with paper towels if wet.

2. On a cutting board, reduce the cooked broccoli into very small pieces.

3. Then area it in a bowl and add the egg. Using a spoon, mix the egg via the broccoli mix as plenty as you could.

4. Heat a few avocado oils in a pan. The oil has to be enough to cowl the bottom, but no extra.

5. Cook on one fire till the cheese at the top of the patty starts off and start to soften and the bottom is crusty brown.

five. Remove from the oil and permit take a seat on a few paper towels for a couple of minutes to soak up the grease, earlier than dishing up. You can serve it topped with an egg or with a dipping sauce.

4. Fourth Week

BREAKFAST

DAY 1	AVOCADO MEAL
	INGREDIENTS FOR AVOCADO MEAL
	1 Avocado dissected into identical 1/2 with the stone removed
	1 Tablespoon of salted butter
	3 Large eggs
	Three slices of bacon cuts into smaller parts
	A pinch of salt
	A pinch of black pepper
	COOKING INSTRUCTIONS
	1. Spoon out maximum of the avocado flesh leaving about half inch across the avocado
	2. On a low warmness, area a frying pan then, upload butter. While the butter is melting destroy the egg into a bowl and beat them adding the black pepper and a pinch of salt
	3. Add the bacon to one quit of the pan and permit them to fry for a couple of minutes without stirring. Then, upload the eggs at the opposite bottom of the pan and blend as they scramble. Within five mins the eggs and bacon ought to be equipped, however if the eggs get

	completed before the bacon you can dispose of the eggs and location it in a bowl four. Then blend the bacon portions and egg in a bowl and scoop it into the avocado bowl, and the meal is ready to be eaten.
DAY 2	THE CAULIFLOWER CARBONARA PAN MEAL INGREDIENTS FOR THE CAULIFLOWER CARBONARA PAN MEAL i. 2.5 cups of frozen riced Cauliflower ii. Eight slices of bacon iii. Six finely chopped garlic cloves iv. 1 Tablespoon of dried Italian Herb seasoning v. 1 / 2 tablespoon of salt vi. 1 / 2 cup of cashew cream (1/4 heavy cream and 1/4 cup of grated parmesan) vii. Two yolks of egg COOKING INSTRUCTIONS 1. Heat a massive frying pan on average warmness 2. Ensure to use a very sharp knife to cut the bacon into slices. When the frying pan is warm, add the bacon into the frying pan four. Cook by using every so often stirring till the bacon is in the main crispy for approximately 6 mins five. Add the finely chopped garlic

6. Stir thoroughly till the garlic begins to show brown

7. Add within the cauliflower rice then salt and dried herbs

8. Stir thoroughly until the rice begins to soften out, and any liquid produced evaporates.

9. Add the cashew creamer, this is the heavy cream, and while it is added you can start to prepare dinner with this creamer. You can then stir till it thickens, well-formed, and creamy. Then you can serve hot to your people.

10. Top the serving with the clean yolk of an egg and blend in. The warmth of the cauliflower will cook dinner the uncooked egg yolk

DAY 3

FLAXSEED CRACKERS

INGREDIENTS FOR FLAXSEED CRACKERS

i. 1 cup of flaxseed food

ii. Three tablespoons of olive oil

iii. Vinegar

iv. one-quarter cup of apple cider

v. half of tablespoon of water

vi. half of tablespoon of sea salt

COOKING INSTRUCTIONS

	1. Get a Container and mix all the ingredients. Mix till properly-shaped then go away it for 20minutes 2. Preheat the oven on 320F convection bake 3. Using a Turner to transfer the flaxseed blend to a sheet of bakery paper then cover with another foil and make it flat four. You can make use of a rolling pin to make it greater flatten till a square shape is shaped, then dispose of the top sheet of the bakery paper and pass the foil at the bottom with the dough on it to a baking pan then pop within the oven and bake within 40-45 mins until the middle is firm. That is when you tab it, it needs to be solid 5. Place it away from the oven and permit it cool to room temperature, then switch the bakery paper with cracker mass to a slicing board and with a big kitchen knife reduce into squares to make your preferred shape.
DAY 4	HEALTHFUL CHICKEN SALAD INGREDIENTS FOR HEALTHFUL CHICKEN SALAD i. 2 cups of Chicken breast portions ii. 2 cups of reduced steamed fresh beans iii. 1/2 cup of self-made mayonnaise iv. 1/2 cup of diced pecans

v. one-quarter cup of diced cilantro

vi. 1/4 cup of basil leaves

vii. 1/4 cup of mint leaves

viii. half tablespoon salt

ix. 1/2 tablespoon of white pepper

COOKING INSTRUCTIONS

1. Cut and dice your herb, pecans and green beans then portions the chicken

2. In a big bowl placed all the elements and mix gently to mix it up

3. Ready to eat

DAY 5	MEDITERRANEAN POKE MIXED WITH AHI TUNA AND CITRUS

MEDITERRANEAN POKE MIXED WITH AHI TUNA AND CITRUS

INGREDIENTS FOR MEDITERRANEAN POKE MIXED WITH AHI TUNA AND CITRUS

i. 8oz Yellow Fin Ahi Tuna fillet

ii. 1 Tablespoon of coconut aminos

iii. Five sprigs cilantro

iv. 1 / 2 Haas avocado

v. Two tablespoons of sesame seeds

vi. 1/4 cup of pili nuts

vii. 1 Tablespoon of sea salt

viii. 1 / 4 ruby red grapefruit

COOKING INSTRUCTIONS

	1. Cut your Ahi Tuna into 1/4-inch cubes and places right into a big bowl 2. Next, add for your coconut aminos, salt, and sesame oil. Mix gently 3, Halve your grapefruit, cuts into exclusive sections then upload them on your bowl 4. Finely chop your cilantro and encompass it right into a bowl 5. Dice your pili nuts, chop your avocado, add it to the bowl and lightly mix to mix the ingredients 6. Divide the Ahi Tuna mix between bowls and decorate with sesame seeds.
DAY 6	TOMATO SALAD, BACON AND EGG INGREDIENTS FOR TOMATO SALAD, BACON AND EGG i. Three slices of bacon ii. one-quarter purple pepper iii. 1/4 Zucchini iv. Two eggs v. Pinch of pepper and salt vi. Three slices of tomatoes vii. One basil leaf viii. 1 Tablespoon of olive oil

	ix. 1 / 2 tablespoon vinegar x. One garlic clove xi. Sprinkle pepper COOKING INSTRUCTIONS 1. Slice the zucchini and crimson pepper 2. Fry the bacon in a small nonstick frying pan till it turns crispy. Place the bacon on a plate. Fry the zucchini and peppers within the bacon fat until it's tender. Sprinkle the pepper and salt over. Put at the plate with the bacon. three. Finely chop the garlic clove and basil leaf. Mix the olive oil, vinegar, basil, garlic, salt, and pepper in a bowl. Add the tomato chopped to the plate and pour the dressing over.
DAY 7	ZOODLES AND AVOCADO CREAM MEAL INGREDIENTS FOR ZOODLES AND AVOCADO CREAM MEAL i. One zucchini ii. half of avocado iii. 20 basil leaves iv. Three brown mushrooms v. 1/5 tablespoon of olive oil vi. One garlic clove vii. 1 Tablespoon of lemon juice

viii. 1/4 tablespoon of salt

COOKING INSTRUCTIONS

1. Cut your zucchini in a spiral shape.

2. Slice the mushrooms into halves.

three. In a stick blender cup, mix the avocado, basil leaves, 1 tablespoon of olive oil, garlic, salt, and lemon juice. Press the on button at the stick blender for approximately 1 minute to permit the combination of the substances for a remarkable creamy and yummy.

4. Add half of the tablespoon of olive oil in a saucepan and prepare dinner the mushrooms until it is smooth, then upload the zucchini noodles and prepare dinner for 1 minute or more until it gets warm.

5. Add the avocado cream and mix the entirety, then serve.

LUNCH

DAY 1	CAULI RICE AND CHICKEN CUTLET
	INGREDIENTS FOR CAULI RICE AND CHICKEN CUTLET
	i. One small cauliflower

ii. Two tablespoon sesame oil

iii. 1 Tablespoon coconut aminos

iv. One egg

v. Four tablespoon almond flour

vi. 1 Tablespoon dashi powder

vii. one-quarter tablespoon salt and pepper

viii. Pinch of salt and pepper

ix. One skinless bird breast

x. 40g beef rinds

xi. Frying oil (refined coconut oil)

COOKING INSTRUCTIONS

1. Dice the riced cauliflower in a part of meals via the use of a cheese grater. In a neat saucepan that you have put on stove, heat the same oil and put the riced cauliflower. Fry for about ten minutes, then start to add the coconut aminos, dashi powder, salt, and pepper then blend properly. Fry till the cauliflower is crunchy and smooth

2. Grind the pork rinds using a meals processor or your palms. Mix the beef rinds with pepper, salt, and almond flour. Break the egg in a bowl, upload it to different elements and whisk the whole thing.3. Chop the fowl breast in 2 lengthways. Sprinkle the pepper and salt on both sides and dip into the whisked egg. Coat the hen with the breading on each quit.

	4. Fry the cutlet in temperature of 150C / 300F preheated oil and fry until the internal temperature of the bird cutlet is 65C /150F. You can serve with the cauli rice.
DAY 2	SHIRATAKI NOODLES AND ASIAN SALAD INGREDIENTS FOR SHIRATAKI NOODLES AND ASIAN SALAD i. Shirataki Noodles (konjac) ii. Two asparagus (40g) iii. 1/2 cup of cucumber (65g) iv. half of tomato (65g) v. One stem cilantro vi. One garlic vii. One egg viii. Two tablespoons of coconut aminos ix. 1/16 red onions (20g) x. 1 Tablespoon fish sauce xi. 1 Tablespoon lemon juice xii. 1 / 2 tablespoon sesame oil xiii. 1/4 tablespoon of salt and pepper xiv. 1/4 tablespoon of warm chili oil COOKING INSTRUCTIONS 1. Place some water in a pot to boil. Put the egg in the

	water and simmer for 7 minutes exactly. Once cooked, do away with the egg and put it in a bowl of ice water. Peel the egg and cut it into four pieces. 2. Wash the shirataki noodles underwater and boil for two minutes. That will really get rid of the smell. In the same pot consist of the asparagus and prepare dinner till tender. Drain the water and allow the noodles and asparagus to settle down. You can smash the noodles into smaller parts. three. Dice the purple onion with a cabbage shredder then reduce the asparagus into 1/2. Chop the tomato, slice the cucumber, cube the cilantro, and finely chop the garlic the use of a garlic crusher. 4. Pour all of the ingredients, at the same time, right into a bowl, then integrate properly. Ensure to serve bloodless.
DAY 3	LETTUCE MEAL INGREDIENT FOR LETTUCE MEAL i. Two lettuce leaves ii. Two chopped bacon iii. 1/4 tomato iv. half avocado v. 1 Tablespoon of mayonnaise

	vi. Two lettuce leaves COOKING INSTRUCTIONS 1. Ensure you start cooking by frying the bacon in a neat and good saucepan until it turns crispy and inviting. 2. Chop the tomato into a few slices, chop the avocado as nicely. three. Use half of tablespoon of mayonnaise over every lettuce leaf and cover with the bacon, tomato, and avocado.
DAY 4	LETTUCE - WRAPPED BURGER INGREDIENTS FOR LETTUCE - WRAPPED BURGER i. 70g grounded pork ii. Two slices of bacon (50g) iii. One large lettuce leaf iv. One slice tomato v. 1 cup of fresh toddler spinach vi. 1 Tablespoon of mayonnaise COOKING INSTRUCTIONS 1. Fry by dipping the bacon in oil that is being heated in a very neat frying pan until its crispy. Form a

	hamburger patty with the ground pork. Then fry within the leftover bacon grease. Cook on both ends until its chefs properly. 2. Add the spinach to the remaining oil within the frying pan and cook till wilted. three. Add the tomato, spinach, mayonnaise, patty and bacon in a big lettuce leaf, fold and make a burger.
DAY 5	**GRILLED COD AND SHRIMPS** **INGREDIENTS FOR GRILLED COD AND SHRIMPS** i. Two cod fillet ii. 1 Tablespoon of lemon juice iii. Two tablespoons of olive oil iv. Two garlic cloves v. Eight cherry tomatoes vi. 200g shrimps vii. 2 stems fresh parsley viii. Two garlic cloves **COOKING INSTRUCTIONS** 1. Finely chop the garlic and parsley. 2. Melt the butter in a pan and encompass the garlic. Cook for few seconds and puts the cod and shrimp in the pan. Add the chopped parsley. Cook the shrimps for

	few mins until it turns orange. Cook the cod for two minutes on every side, be cautious not to interrupt it aside while turning it over. Include the tomatoes to the pan and fry with the shrimps for about one minute till it's far soft. three. Add the lemon juice. Then it's far set to be eaten.
DAY 6	ARUGULA CAESAR SALAD AND VEGETABLES INGREDIENTS FOR ARUGULA CAESAR SALAD AND VEGETABLES i. Three leaves of iceberg lettuce ii. Two asparagus iii. 40g arugula iv. Four broccoli florets v. 5-6 slices cucumber vi. half of avocado vii. 1 / 2 tomato One part of Caesar dressing COOKING INSTRUCTIONS 1. Place some water to boil and cook dinner the broccoli and asparagus until it is smooth 2. Shred the arugula and iceberg lettuce and vicinity into a bowl 3. Chop the avocado, cucumber, and tomato. Then

	positioned the entirety into a plate and cowl with the dressing
DAY 7	FLUFFY OMELET AND VEGETABLES INGREDIENTS i. half zucchini ii. 1 / 2 cup of fresh spinach iii. half of small cucumber iv. One hard-boiled egg v. 1 serving basil Vinaigrette COOKING INSTRUCTIONS 1. Using a cabbage shredder, slice the zucchini and cucumber thinly 2. Slice the spinach and reduce the egg into four three. Place everything right into a plate and pour the dressing

DINNER

DAY 1	ARUGULA SALAD WITH BASIL VINAIGRETTE INGREDIENTS FOR ARUGULA SALAD WITH BASIL VINAIGRETTE i. 40g arugula ii. five to six slices of cucumber iii. 1 / 2 tomato

	iv. Two slices prosciutto v. Three broccoli florets vi. 1 serving basil Vinaigrette COOKING INSTRUCTIONS 1. When water is boiling upload the broccoli to it. Cook, until it's far soft and cool, relaxed beneath bloodless water. 2. Mix all the elements in a cooking container, and you're set.
DAY 2	BROCCOLI AND ROSEMARY CHICKEN INGREDIENTS FOR BROCCOLI AND ROSEMARY CHICKEN i. One boneless bird leg ii. one-quarter tablespoon of salt iii. half of tablespoon of rosemary iv. 1 Tablespoon of olive oil v. 1/3 broccoli head vi. one-quarter tablespoon of black pepper vii. Two tablespoons of water COOKING INSTRUCTIONS 1. Cut the chicken leg into bite-length pieces, then sprinkle salt and pepper on pinnacle of it. Separate the broccoli into florets.

	2. In a cast-iron pan, permit the olive oil to get heated, and upload the hen to the rosemary. Fry for three minutes to crisp up the chook pores and skin and turn the bird around. Then continue to add the prepared broccoli florets, with that you can prepare dinner for two minutes blending the components, then inside the water, cowl it and allow the steam of the water to cook the broccoli for 2 minutes. Then scoop it and serve to your people.
DAY 3	ROASTED ROSEMARY PORK INGREDIENTS FOR ROASTED ROSEMARY PORK i. 500g boneless roast beef ii. 1 Tablespoon of olive oil iii. 1 Tablespoon of salt iv. 1 Tablespoon of black pepper v. 1 Tablespoon of rosemary COOKING INSTRUCTIONS 1 Preheat the oven in a temperature of 200C/400F. 2. Gently rubdown the salt, black pepper, salt, and rosemary into the beef roast, then placed it on a baking tray wrapped in bakery paper. 3. Put it within the oven and cook for one hour. Remove

	it, and permit it cool for 5 to ten mins. Slice and serve.
DAY 4	KALE BEEF AND VEGETABLES WRAPPED
	INGREDIENTS FOR KALE BEEF AND VEGETABLES WRAPPED
	i. half of avocado
	ii. 1 / 2 tomato
	iii. One portion of Caesar dressing
	iv. One massive kale leaf
	v. 1/8 purple onion
	vi. 100g thinly sliced beef
	vii. one-quarter tablespoon of pepper, salt, and garlic powder
	viii. 1 Tablespoon of olive oil
	COOKING INSTRUCTIONS
	1. Trim the stem of the kale leaf cautiously to enable you to roll the leaf to make a sandwich.
	2. Chop the avocado, tomato, and red onion.
	three. Place a saucepan with olive oil on a cooker and include the sliced red meat into the pan. Sprinkle the garlic powder, pepper, and salt and cook very well for 1 to 2 minutes.
	four. Scoop the Caesar dressing over the complete leaf. On one of the ceases, upload all of the toppings and roll the leaf into a wrap carefully. You can employ the

	aluminum foil to maintain it from rolling away.
DAY 5	EGG IN MINI SKILLET INGREDIENTS FOR EGG IN MINI SKILLET i. Two slices of bacon ii. 1 / 2 avocado iii. Two eggs iv. 1 / 2 tomato v. One okra vi. Three boiled broccoli vii. Sprinkle pepper, parsley, and salt COOKING INSTRUCTIONS 1. Fry the bacon till it is crispy in a mini skillet of 6 inches. Chop the bacon into bits. Dice the avocado and tomato and slice the okra into some portions 2. Using the same mini skillet, crack the eggs open into the bacon grease, cowl, and cook dinner on low heat till it cooks properly. Top it with the bacon bits, avocado, broccoli, okra, and tomato. Sprinkle salt, parsley, and pepper over it,
DAY 6	MUSHROOMS, BROCCOLI AND BACON MEAL INGREDIENTS FOR MUSHROOMS, BROCCOLI

	AND BACON MEAL i. 8og of broccoli ii. Four brown mushrooms iii. Three portions of bacon iv. one-quarter tablespoon of salt v. half tablespoon of rosemary vi. one-quarter tablespoon of garlic powder vii. A pinch of black pepper COOKING INSTRUCTIONS 1. Boil little water in a pot and cook dinner the broccoli until it is soft. 2. Sprinkle salt over the bacon pieces and reduce into 1cm peeps. 3. Cut the mushrooms into six portions. 4. Fry the bacon in a pan for one minute and include the mushrooms. Add the rosemary to the broccoli, then blend the entirety, sprinkle the garlic powder, and black pepper on it.
DAY 7	RADISHES AND ROSEMARY SHRIMPS INGREDIENTS FOR RADISHES AND ROSEMARY SHRIMPS i. Five radishes ii. 1 Tablespoon olive oil iii. 1 Tablespoon of rosemary

	iv. Ten shrimps v. Three broccoli florets vi. half tablespoon salt and pepper COOKING INSTRUCTIONS 1. Boil some water in a pot and upload the broccoli then cook dinner until it tenders. 2. Put a frying pan with olive oil on a cooker to heat it, then include the radishes to an aspect and the shrimps to every other aspect, then sprinkle the salt, rosemary, and pepper and cook for few mins. The radishes should be crunchy and soft, and you must make certain the shrimps turn orange. Three. Put the whole thing in a plate and experience it.

DESSERT

DAY 1	LOW CARB BREAD INGREDIENTS FOR LOW CARB BREAD i. Four tablespoons of easily grounded almond meal ii. one-quarter tablespoon of baking soda iii. One huge egg iv. Two tablespoons of water v. Two tablespoons of olive oil

	vi. 1 / 4 tablespoon of salt COOKING INSTRUCTIONS 1. In a shallow small microwave-secure container, whisk the flour, salt, and baking soda together. 2. Make a hollow inside the center and destroy an egg open into it, then whisk well. Add inside the olive oil and water at the same time as blending. three. When it forms very well, start making large circles together with your fork to comprise the flour blend. four. Mix thoroughly, including the edges and sides, then use a spatula to make certain it mixes flawlessly. five. Tap the bowl down on the counter to ensure the combination settle. 6. Microwave for ninety seconds on high heat or heat until the center is properly cooked. 7. If you're baking it, employ a greased glass dish and bake at 325F convection for 20 mins, then use a spatula across the facets to separate it from the container. eight. Pop right into a toaster for three-4 mins until it's miles crispy and geared up to eat.
DAY 2	THE MEDITERRANEAN ALMOND BUTTER BURGER INGREDIENTS FOR THE MEDITERRANEAN ALMOND BUTTER BURGER

	i. Two tablespoons of grounded turkey ii. 1 Tablespoon of apple cider iii. Vinegar iv. One large egg v. half cup of almond butter crunchy and unsweetened vi. 1 Tablespoon of black pepper vii. 1 Tablespoon of fish sauce viii. 1 Tablespoon of turmeric ix. 1 / 2 tablespoon of garlic salt COOKING INSTRUCTIONS 1. Start by way of preheating the oven till it gets to 400F. 2. Mix all the listed ingredients above right into a massive bowl until well-formed, then gently grease a large baking sheet. three. Shape into ten patties like four oz every then area at the baking sheet. four. Bake for 20-25 mins.
DAY 3	MEDITERRANEAN MEAL WITH GREEN SAUCE INGREDIENTS FOR MEDITERRANEAN MEAL WITH GREEN SAUCE i. 1 cup of child spinach ii. 1 cup of arugula

iii. 1 cup of parsley

iv. Five medium of garlic cloves

v. Five tablespoons of hemp hearts

vi. 1 cup of olive oil

vii. Five slices bacon

viii. Two eggs

ix. 20 asparagus guidelines

x. Salt

xi. Pepper

COOKING INSTRUCTIONS

1. To make a green sauce integrate child spinach, parsley, garlic cloves, arugula, and olive oil right into a blender and mix the components on low speed until it's far properly-fashioned and easy and set aside.

2. On a sheet pan, arrange your bacon chops into rings and prepare it into circles.

three. Pop the sheet pan into the oven then set to a temperature of 320F. When the oven is at excessive temperature, take away the sheet pan from the oven and suit the four asparagus suggestions into every bacon ring.

4. Move your bacon rings together if essential after which spoil two eggs in among them.

five. Add your already made green sauce, sprinkle little pepper and salt and go back to the oven for 20minutes.

	6. Remove from the oven and enjoy!
DAY 4	ASPARAGUS, SAUCE AND AVOCADO BOAT MEAL INGREDIENTS FOR ASPARAGUS, SAUCE AND AVOCADO BOAT MEAL i. Asparagus, sausage and avocado boat ii. 60g sausage iii. 1 or 2 asparagus iv. 1 Tablespoon olive oil v. half of avocado vi. 70g Tuna vii. 1/4 cup of wilted spinach viii. 1 Tablespoon of mayonnaise ix. Pinch salt and pepper COOKING INSTRUCTIONS 1. Place a small frying pan on fireplace to warmth the olive oil and fry the sausages and asparagus until its chefs well then transfer to a plate. 2. Spoon out the inner of the avocado and put it in a bowl with the Tuna, mayonnaise, wilted spinach and salt and pepper. Put the avocado shell with it and area it on a plate.

DAY 5	VEGETABLES BROCHETTES AND CHICKEN INGREDIENTS FOR VEGETABLES BROCHETTES AND CHICKEN i. One boneless bird leg (300g) ii. four Asparagus iii. 1 Tablespoon of rosemary iv. Ten cherry tomatoes v. Five garlic cloves vi. half of tablespoon of onion powder vii. 1 Tablespoon of salt and pepper viii. 1 Tablespoon of olive oil ix. 1 Tablespoon lemon juice from a lemon x. One huge Asian COOKING INSTRUCTIONS 1. Preheat the oven to 210C / 420F. 2. Chop the chook leg into biteable portions. Slice the lengthy green onion into 12 to 14 pieces. Then cut the asparagus into 4. 3. Combine all the substances into a cooking bowl and blend. Skewer the vegetables and fowl on the brochettes. 4. Place within the oven and bake for 20 mins.

DAY 6	SESAME SALAD AND CHICKEN BROCHETTES INGREDIENTS FOR SESAME SALAD AND CHICKEN BROCHETTES i. Three chook and vegetable brochettes ii. Three lettuce leaves iii. One tomato slice iv. One portion of sesame dressing v. 1/4 avocado COOKING INSTRUCTIONS 1. Cut the lettuce into portions size biteable. Scoop out the avocado flesh and cube it, chop the tomato into few portions. Add the sesame dressing and coat thoroughly. 2. Add the brochettes to a plate with the salad and experience!
DAY 7	PORK OMELET AND SPINACH INGREDIENTS FOR PORK OMELET AND SPINACH i. One sausage ii. 1 cup of sparkling spinach iii. 1/4 crimson pepper iv. Two garlic cloves v. Two tablespoons of olive oil vi. 1/ 4 tablespoon of pepper, garlic powder, and salt

vii. 1/4 tablespoon of parsley

viii. Six eggs

COOKING INSTRUCTIONS

1. Crush the sausage. Chop the purple pepper and finely chop the garlic.

2. In a massive nonstick frying pan, prepare dinner the sausage and add the olive oil. Add the crimson pepper, spinach, and garlic to the pan and cook dinner for 1 or 2 minutes until it is soft.

three. Break the eggs open in a massive bowl, add the spices and combine with a whisk for two minutes.

four. Pour the battered egg to the pan, then cowl and permit it to prepare dinner on a low warmth for 4 to five minutes.

5. When the pinnacle of the omelet is ready, slide the omelet to a plate and reduce into two you may eat 1/2 nowadays and the opposite the next day.

SNACK

DAY 1	CHICKEN GRILLED THIGH WITH ZUCCHINI SALAD

CHICKEN GRILLED THIGH WITH ZUCCHINI SALAD

INGREDIENTS FOR CHICKEN GRILLED THIGH WITH ZUCCHINI SALAD

i. 1/4 Zucchini

ii. 1/4 purple pepper

iii. Five basil leaves

iv. One garlic clove

v. One fowl thigh with a skin of (75g)

vi. 50g Swiss chard

vii. 1/2 tablespoon of salt and pepper

viii. 1 Tablespoon of olive oil

ix. 1 Tablespoon of vinegar

x. one-quarter tomato

COOKING INSTRUCTIONS

1. Using a peeler, peel the zucchini in a lengthwise shape to make lengthy ribbons. Cut the red pepper in 1/2. Dice the tomato. Slice the Swiss chard. Finely chop the basil leaves and garlic cloves.

2. Mix all of the above substances with olive oil, salt, pepper, and vinegar together in a bowl and location it on a plate.

3. Spray the salt and pepper over the hen thigh. Preheat the oil in a cast-iron pan and location the hen breast skin aspect down and prepare dinner till it is miles crispy.

	Flip it around, cook a few more mins until nicely cooked, then area on the plate with the salad.
DAY 2	GRILLED SALMON AND GREEN BEANS AND RADISHES INGREDIENTS FOR GRILLED SALMON AND GREEN BEANS AND RADISHES i. 150g of salmon fillet ii. 3 Tablespoon of olive oil iii. one-quarter tablespoon of salt, black pepper, and dill iv. 1 Tablespoon of lemon juice v. 1 Tablespoon of rosemary vi. Five radishes vii. Pinch of salt, garlic powder, and pepper viii. One garlic clove ix. 50g green beans COOKING INSTRUCTIONS 1. Rub the salmon with oil, salt, pepper and dill. 2. Place a nonstick frying pan carefully and cook on both aspects for two to 3 minutes until it's miles perfectly cooked via. Once nicely cooked, add the lemon juice on top of the salmon 3. Finely chop the garlic clove. Place the green beans to a boil and prepare dinner for 5 to six mins. Take out of

	the water into a pan accompany the olive oil and the finely chopped garlic. Sprinkle the salt and pepper over it and prepare dinner in the frying pan until the garlic receives crunchy. four. Put a frying pan with olive oil on a cooker to heat the olive oil, then include the rosemary and radishes. Then mix cook for 4-five mins till it is miles crispy. Sprinkle the salt and pepper on it once more.
DAY 3	COCONUT FLOUR PORRIDGE INGREDIENTS FOR COCONUT FLOUR PORRIDGE i. 2 tablespoons coconut flour ii. 2 tablespoons golden flax meal iii. 3/four cup water iv. Pinch of salt v. 1 large egg beaten vi. 2 teaspoons butter or ghee vii. 1 tablespoon heavy cream or coconut milk viii. 1 tablespoon Low carb brown sugar or your favorite sweetener Instructions 1. Start by measuring the first four substances right into a saucepan or a small pot. Allow it to warmness for approximately 5mins and stir. When it starts to simmer,

flip it down to medium-low and whisk till it starts off evolved to thicken.

2. Remove the coconut flour porridge from heat and add the crushed egg, half at a time, even as whisking the mixture continuously. Place it back on the heat and keep whisking until the porridge thickens.

three. Remove the pan from the warmth and maintain to whisk for about 30 seconds before including the butter, cream and sweetener.

4. Garnish it along with your favored toppings.

MEDITERRANEAN BAKED OMELET

INGREDIENTS FOR MEDITERRANEAN BAKED OMELET

i. half lb. Browned and crumbled sausage

ii. 8 massive eggs

iii. 1/2 cup heavy whipping cream

iv. 1 cup shredded Cheddar cheese

v. Salt, pepper, and other seasonings, to flavor good

Instructions

1. Preheat oven to 380°F. Spray a 7x11-inch baking dish with non-stick cooking spray.

2. Place the cooked and crumbled sausage flippantly within the prepared pan.

	3. In a big bowl, whisk the eggs, heavy cream, cheese, and any preferred seasonings until they're nicely combined. Pour the egg combination frivolously over the sausage. four. Bake for half-hour or until the edges start to brown. Then your Mediterranean omelet is prepared to be served.
DAY 4	CHEESY BACON OMELET INGREDIENTS FOR CHEESY BACON OMELET i. 3 Large Eggs ii. 30 g Cheddar Cheese Grated iii. 2 Slices bacon Instructions 1. Heat a frying pan to medium-high heat, wait until you can experience the heat by soaring your hand five centimeters above the pan. 2. Place the bacon in the pan and prepare dinner till crispy. three. In an everyday bowl, whisk the eggs. 4. Remove the bacon along with as a good deal grease as possible. Pour it in the whisked eggs. five. Cook for approximately 3-four minutes, area the cheese and bacon on one half of the Omelet and turn one

	side over onto the cheese and bacon. Cook for every other 1-2 minutes.
DAY 5	MEDITERRANEAN FATHEAD PIZZA INGREDIENTS FOR MEDITERRANEAN FATHEAD PIZZA i. 1 half of cup Mozzarella cheese (shredded) ii. 2 tbsp Cream cheese (reduce into cubes) iii. 2 large Egg (beaten) iv. 1/3 cup Coconut flour v. One out of pepperoni, peppers, cherry tomatoes, olives, floor/mince red meat, mushrooms, herbs. Instructions 1. Preheat your oven to 425 levels F (218 tiers C). Start to line a baking sheet, pizza pan with the necessary parchment paper. 2. Mix the diced mozzarella and cubed cream cheese in a massive bowl. Microwave for ninety seconds, stirring halfway through. Stir once more at the stop till nicely incorporated. three. Stir inside the crushed eggs and coconut flour. You must ensure that you knead the flour with your hands until a dough form. If the dough turns into hard before fully combined, you could microwave for 10-15

seconds to melt it.

4. Spread the dough onto the covered baking pan to 1/4" or 1/3" thickness, the use of your arms or a rolling pin over a piece of parchment. However, the rolling pin works better when you have one. You must ensure to use a toothpick or the tinge of your spoon or fork to poke lots of holes all through the crust to prevent bubbling and to make sure it cooks flippantly.

five. Bake for six minutes. Poke more holes in any locations wherein you notice bubbles forming. Bake for three-7 extra mins, till golden brown.

6. Once cooked, cast off from the oven and add all the toppings you want. Make positive any meat that you'll be adding inside the topping is already cooked as this time it goes back into the oven simply to warmness up the toppings and melt the cheese. Bake again at 220C/425F for simply 5 minutes.

| DAY 6 | LOADED CAULIFLOWER CASSEROLE |
| | INGREDIENTS FOR LOADED CAULIFLOWER CASSEROLE |

i. 1-pound cauliflower

ii. 4 oz bitter cream

iii. 1 cup cheddar cheese (grated or shredded)

iv. 2 slices bacon cooked and crumbled

	v. 2 tablespoons chives snipped
	vi. 3 tablespoons butter
	vii. one-quarter teaspoon garlic powder
	viii. Salt and black pepper
	Instructions
	1. To begin with, cut the cauliflower into florets, then placed them right into a microwave-safe bowl. Add two tablespoons of water and cover with dangle film.
	2. Add the cauliflower to a meals processor and system till it turns into fluffy. Add the butter, garlic powder, and buttercream, then technique until it resembles the consistency of mashed potatoes.
	three. Top the loaded cauliflower with the final cheese, closing chives and bacon. Put lower back into the microwave to melt the cheese or place the cauliflower under the broiler for a couple of minutes.
DAY 7	BROCCOLI FRITTERS WITH CHEDDAR CHEESE INGREDIENTS FOR BROCCOLI FRITTERS WITH CHEDDAR CHEESE i. 1 small broccoli head or 1/2 large one ii. 1 egg (beaten) iii. A handful of grated cheddar cheese iv. 2 Tbsp oat fiber or almond flour, or powdered beef rinds

v. 1Tbsps avocado oil or any of your favored oil

Instructions

1. First, loosely chop your broccoli and then steam gently for a few minutes till it's far tender. Drain any excess water and dry with paper towels if wet.

2. On a cutting board, reduce the cooked broccoli into very small pieces.

3. Then area it in a bowl and add the egg. Using a spoon, mix the egg via the broccoli mix as plenty as you could.

4. Heat a few avocado oils in a pan. The oil has to be enough to cowl the bottom, but no extra.

5. Cook on one fire till the cheese at the top of the patty starts off and start to soften and the bottom is crusty brown.

five. Remove from the oil and permit take a seat on a few paper towels for a couple of minutes to soak up the grease, earlier than dishing up. You can serve it topped with an egg or with a dipping sauce.

CONCLUSION

Mediterranean food is known to be healthy and good for extending human lifespan, having fit and healthy mind. Well, we may not know for sure what the future of human health and longevity will be, but we can assume and predict it. It is known that food high in too much carbohydrate and unhealthy calories increase the risk of heart disease, stroke and kidney failure, but only a few books have examined how Mediterranean foods can lower those risks and effects longevity or increases someone lifespan. Other things like having green trees in the neighborhood, eating green leaves, seafoods, exposing ourselves to consumption of wheat, tofa, spinach and other grains with less red meat but more fish like salmon, mackerel, tuna are linked to longevity, youthful look and this book has done justice to that. Mediterranean food is probably the most essential secret to weight loss and a necessary key to having a perfect shape and good look. Another secret is we should take many antioxidants in high doses – I believe that the content of this book which is primarily centered on Mediterranean foods, if rightly applied, could significantly improve the future of human health and longevity, as well as advances one's weight lose plan.

Good luck!